They Grow in Silence

They Grow in Silence:

Understanding Deaf Children and Adults

Second Edition

Edited by

Eugene D. Mindel, M.D.
McCay Vernon, Ph.D.

☐ *Published for the National Association for the Deaf* ☐

**COLLEGE-HILL
PRESS**

A College-Hill Publication
Little, Brown and Company
Boston/Toronto/San Diego

HV
2391
.T44
1987

College-Hill Press
A Division of
Little, Brown and Company (Inc.)
34 Beacon Street
Boston, Massachusetts 02108

Library of Congress Cataloging in Publication Data
Main entry under title:

They grow in silence.
Includes index.
1. Children, Deaf. 2. Deafness. 3. Deafness —
Psychological aspects. 4. Deaf — Means of communication.
5. Children, Deaf — Family relationships. I. Mindel,
Eugene D. II. Vernon, McCay.
HV2391.T44   1987   362.4'2'088054   86-21638
ISBN 0-316-57422-8

ISBN 0-316-57422-8

Printed in the United States of America.

Contents

DEDICATION

Most readers of this book never knew personally nor have heard the name, Fred Schreiber, the first executive director of the National Association of the Deaf, a position he held until his death in 1979. Germaine to this writing, Fred rescued the first edition of this book from a premature demise.

"They Grow In Silence" was originally to be published by the subsidiary of a large textbook concern under the editorship of Joe McMenamin, who had become acquainted with the special needs of deaf children through his personal friends, Mr. and Mrs. Marion Reis, also editors. The manuscript had progressed to galley proofs when the publisher, in a policy dispute with the parent company, resigned voluntarily. Joe was forced to resign. His replacement called to say that he believed our book would not even sell an initial run of 3,000 copies. Soon thereafter we contacted N.A.D. to solicit their interest. Within a month, we had a new publisher and I a new friend. Fourteen years and over 35,000 copies distributed worldwide have well erased the pain of that rejection, but not that of the loss of Fred.

Fred Schreiber was one of those people you know you really know soon after you meet. Thinking back on the years between 1971 and 1979, between telephone calls, a few exchanges of letters and a handful of brief meetings, I spent in sum no more than a few hours with that kind, punchy, gifted and visionary administrator. His bigger than life quality made those few hours seem like many more. In Fred's company one always was with Fred; he'd put his full creative capacity into every moment.

Especially endearing to me was a quality Fred shared with my father, Sidney Mindel, to whom the first edition was dedicated — they both could talk to anyone and both usually delighted in doing so. I am sure that observed quality contributed in no small measure to my choosing psychiatry as a profession and, in 1966, accepting an opportunity to work in deafness with my co-editor and now long time friend McCay Vernon and with Roy Grinker, Sr., under whom I trained in psychiatry.* Once beginning that position, I quickly learned that the joy derived from talking with other people could not be taken for granted. Worse, I further learned, legions of educators, parents and others had been, for one hundred years, subjecting deaf children to a kind of arduous education that most often poorly served their communication handicap. These people believed there was something inherently wrong in allowing deaf children to use their natural language, the language of sign. The strident tone of that volume minimally expressed my outrage and barely reflected the heat in the many arguments (some more ugly than I care to remember) I'd found myself a participant in having seen the wrongheadedness of that view.

As will be documented within the pages that follow, this country, since the publication of the first edition, has seen a momentous shift away from an oralist dominated American deaf education establishment to a large scale incorporation of total communication methodologies. Enough good solid research has been conducted and validated to substantiate the many commonsense beliefs set forth in the first edition.

So many developments in medicine, psychiatry, psychology, audiology, education and psycholinguistics have occurred that undertaking a complete rewrite of "They Grow In Silence" without additional contributors would have been impossible. I am honored to include here original articles by distinguished collaborators along with revised chapters from the first edition.

More than ever, with the weight of solid open-minded observation and research in the years since 1972, I am convinced that the only reasonable and fair educational methods for deaf children incorporate Total Communication into school, home and commu-

---

*This association is described by Dr. Grinker in his introduction to the first edition.

nity. Surviving in a chaotic world mandates that our children are offered the largest communication repertory possible — to exercise and enjoy their inalienable right to the freedom of speech.

Some time early in my work in deafness, I met the Untermyer family of River Woods. Abraham was perhaps 2 years old. Soon after learning he was deaf, all members of his family began using Total Communication in all conversations where he was present. Often his parents and his older siblings (they were many years older) would kneel before him to ensure his ability to see their signs, to know their minds. Younger Alexander learned to sign as he learned to speak.

Abraham's mother, Ethel, reviewed and generously commented on the original manuscript of the first edition. The following quote from her comments was included in the section on semantics in Chapter 5 ("Social, Educational and Language Development," p. 53).

> Last summer, our son's summer-program teacher came to our house for a sign-language class. She is deaf; her finance, also deaf, was to teach the lesson. Abraham exhibited the same delight, disappointment, competition, and curiosity as our hearing children have when they learn that here was his teacher's boyfriend to whom she was to be married. We found him a delightful, bright, and mischievous guy. Abraham sized-up this competitor for his teacher's affection, and sensed an important part of the young man's personality, calling out to him in sign-language, "You're a little devil!"

This quote demonstrated the burgeoning subtlety in Abraham's expressive capacity gifted to him by his dedicated family. In 1982, upon the death of his grandmother, Abraham wrote a poem that was included on the announcement of her death. Fred Schreiber was a personal idol of Abraham Untermeyer. It is therefore fitting that I close this dedication to Fred by quoting that poem,* a personal statement of love for a grandmother, a testament to the unending creativity of the human spirit, liberated and articulate.

---

*Reprinted with permission of the author.

she spoke german
    so she could speak in germany.
she spoke english
    so she could speak in the United States
she spoke sign language
    so she could speak to a grandchild.
i am the grandchild.
she spoke with ease to me
    (even when things were down)
not afraid to speak to
someone who is different
from most people.
today,
i spread my hands wide open
and
carry the coffin
containing her and her hands,
                retired.

Eugene D. Mindel
Wilmette, Illinois
1986

Foreword to First Edition

The history of the involvement of the Institute for Psychosomatic and Psychiatric Research and Training of the Michael Reese Hospital and Medical Center in the psychosocial problems of deaf persons is somewhat complicated, but worth sketching. During the latter part of World War II, I was stationed at an air force rehabilitation center as chief of professional services. Stationed at a nearby air base, a young otologist, Dr. Robert Henner, also from Michael Reese Hospital, frequently visited me to talk about psychological problems in his field.

When we returned to our civilian duties, Dr. Henner raised funds and organized a Hearing and Speech Center just as I was planning and designing a Psychiatric Institute; both were opened at Michael Reese Hospital in 1951. Dr. Henner constantly pleaded with me for psychiatric help in his work. Unfortunately, we could spare no psychiatrist because we were attempting to build up a body of professionals in the decade of the 1950's for a just emerging field. Dr. Henner died in 1960 before we could cooperate with this pioneer who understood the immense psychological and psychiatric problems associated with deafness.

In 1965, Dr. McCay Vernon became director of a planning survey at DePaul University to determine the possibility of a coordinated training program for professionals interested in working with persons handicapped by defects in speech and hearing. About the same time, Michael Reese received a donation for a free-standing Hearing and Speech Center to be named after the late Mr. David Siegel, in which the Dr. Robert Henner Hearing and Speech Center was to be the Diagnostic and Therapy section. Frequent conferences with members of the Social and Rehabilitation Service of the Department of Health, Education and Welfare (HEW) and others, a visit to the pioneering state mental hospital at Rockland,

New York, where Drs. Alschuler and Ranier had initiated a unit for the study of deaf psychotics, stirred our own interest. We were able to obtain a three-year grant for the support of our work through the cooperation of Miss Mary Switzer and Drs. William Usdane and Boyce Williams. The grant was timed so that our pilot studies would be completed approximately when the Siegel Institute would be ready. The report of our work has been published: *Psychiatric Diagnosis Therapy and Research on the Psychotic Deaf* (supported by Department of Health, Education and Welfare Social Rehabilitation Grant Number RD-2407-S, Final Report, September 1, 1969 — Institute for Psychosomatic and Psychiatric Research and Training, Michael Reese Hospital and Medical Center, Chicago).

We were fortunate to have in our working group not only professionals working with deaf adults* but also Dr. Eugene D. Mindel, a child psychiatrist, and Dr. Vernon, a clinical psychologist, who were interested in working with deaf children and their families. This book is the result of their labors and contains not only the data from their investigations but also ideas, suggestions, and conclusions about educational processes important for the families and professionals working with deaf children: pediatricians, psychologists, psychiatrists, social workers, and teachers.

An inadequate understanding of the problems of the deaf abounds in the literature and the pronouncements of professionals, especially educators. The deaf are not dumb in the sense of having lesser or poor capacity for abstraction, for intellectual development, or education. They are indeed handicapped, but made worse by biased concepts of teaching motivated toward maintaining traditional methods encrusted in professional "establishments."

A concerted effort should be directed toward the enlightenment of the families of deaf children to facilitate opportunities for proper education before critical periods are reached, after which adequate education is difficult if at all possible. So many family and marital problems need to be understood: the stress of the deaf child on the family, grandparents' interference, denial of deafness, rationalizations, hostility, and confused or delayed decisions. The natural impact of the discovery of deafness is shock, hostility, guilt, empathic coddling, social isolation, et cetera. It is only when grief,

---

*D. Rothstein, M.D., G. Joosten, M.D., Harry Easton, Ph.D., J.D. Koh, Ph.D., L.L. Collums, M.A., and a number of consultants and technicians.

anger, guilt, and helplessness are resolved that steps are taken to facilitate the teaching of adequate means of communications: manual (signing) plus whatever oral systems are appropriate.

The wide variety of reactions depend on the personality of the parents, the cause of deafness (hereditary, measles, Rh+ factor, prematurity, et cetera) and the degree of deafness. Therefore, early examination for brain damage and early audiological studies are necessary. When the results are known, families can be helped through individual and group therapy and the children dealt with by appropriate psychological and educational methods. Thereby behavioral disturbances that could cripple the deaf child for all of his life can be avoided, and the family can be at peace with itself.

The authors discuss all these problems in detail. In language understandable to the average family, they present cogent arguments for their recommendations and thereby contribute a significant optimistic prediction for the deaf child to grow into a healthy adult who can work well and not underachieve, love well, play well, and socialize with his peers and continue to be optimistic for a good life. This important book may stir angry controversy among those who traditionally fight for unproven assertions, but it tells a story for those who really want to know.

Roy R. Grinker, Sr., M.D.

Director of the Institute
Professor of Psychiatry
Michael Reese Hospital
and Medical Center
Chicago, Illinois

Preface to First Edition

In the spring of 1966, when the Project for the Deaf was in the planning stage at Michael Reese Hospital, Dr. Vernon and I met. Dr. Vernon, then at the University of Illinois, was hired as the planning director for the project; subsequently he became project director. I was completing two years active duty as a Naval Medical Officer. Our first meeting was to discuss my future role as child psychiatrist for the project, and to arrange sign language tutoring for my wife and myself.

I had already become acquainted with the deaf community while still in medical school. With two fellow junior medical students, I worked in the infirmary at Gallaudet College, Washington, D.C., the world's only college exclusively for the deaf. It cannot be said that it was a thoroughly sophisticating experience, for it was only after 1966 that I became aware of the full consequences of deafness. The experience at Gallaudet did serve, however, to help master the initial awkwardness that hearing people experience with deaf people, and I learned fingerspelling and some sign language.

During the ensuing eight years, I never stopped thinking about that experience. I had a recurrent dream in which I met a deaf person and conversed using finger spelling.* A few times, there were actual attempts to use these limited skills, but real understanding or closeness with deaf persons was never achieved. The reasons for this failure have only become clear in the last three years, and form much of the thesis of this work.

---

*I have since discovered that it is not uncommon for people who are attempting to learn a new language to have dreams in which they are conversing in the new language, rather than their native language. This was discovered during discussions of language development with first year residents in a child psychiatry seminar which I conducted at the Illinois State Psychiatric Institute, 1969-1970.

(continued)

While in psychiatric training, my thoughts about deaf people achieved greater definition. Since spoken language in human beings is so significant in establishing relationships, what could the effects be on mental development of not having a fully developed verbal language capacity? And beyond this, what changes take place in personality consequent to this lack? But time was short then and these questions could not be carried into an investigation.

The establishment of the Project for the Deaf in September, 1966, offered the opportunity for such an investigation. It brought together a group of people with somewhat diverse backgrounds but united by a common interest: to help deaf people through seeking a better understanding of their development and problems. Throughout the project, the distillate of many hours of discussions was always the same basic issues. Of these, perhaps the most fundamental is: *If communication difficulty strikes at the heart of the deaf person's plight, why do so many still advocate the use of a method of communication with so many inherent difficulties?* Beyond this, why do passions rise so high when these issues are discussed? For those who have come into work with deaf people without prior commitments to a method, the compelling logic of the problems leads to questioning. Those in the field have so frequently lost all perspective that discussion is impossible.

Some of the traditional controversy confusing and alienating parents and professional workers has been further complicated by a misunderstanding of the word *deafness*. To some, it implies total inability to hear. To others, it means a failure to understand the spoken word immediately. Some virtually deny the existence of deafness and employ the euphemism "hearing impaired." We have found it most meaningful to define deafness as *a loss of hearing*

The residents of that group came from diverse cultural backgrounds. Apparently, as the individual becomes more familiar and comfortable in using a new language — in this case, English — the dreams in which the individual is speaking English diminish in frequency or disappear altogether.

Such experiences suggest to the psychoanalyst or the psychoanalytically oriented psychiatrist the process of dream work operating to overcome difficult and anxiety producing circumstances inherent in adjustment to a new country and new language. A similar phenomenon was apparently operating in my case. The unfamiliar community and language in this case was manual communication and the deaf community. Since working more actively with deaf individuals and becoming more comfortable in the use of manual communication, I have not again had such dreams. Dream analysis beyond the level at which dream fragment is presented would, in each individual, reveal the deeper nature of the importance of communication to him.

sufficiently severe to render an understanding of conversational speech impossible in most situations with or without a hearing aid. In this book, the phrase "severe and profound deafness" derives from this definition.

Although a child may perceive a drum beat, respond to a shout, or look up at an airplane passing overhead, he is psychologically, educationally, and socially deaf if he cannot understand speech. Destructive confusion and controversy has grown from a simple failure to realize that sound perception for random nonspeech noises does not allow an understanding of speech. Deafness so defined seems clear; it sounds logical and too obvious to need special explanation. The current condition of the rehabilitation commitment for the deaf shows that far more than simple definitions are needed. Common sense has been struck down by nonsense.

Over the first two years of the project, Dr. Vernon and I spent many hours discussing the various related issues. More and more, the necessity for a comprehensive statement on deafness and its ramifications grew obvious. The communication controversy must be considered in the whole context of family and community. Important issues are so diverse, their interrelationships so knotty, that brief, sometimes heated discussions almost never lead to resolution. Thus, around the middle of 1969, the idea for this book was born. There seemed only one appropriate way to consider all aspects of the problem — unite them between the covers of a book.

The book was initiated as a cooperative effort and has remained so throughout. Dr. Vernon's seventeen years of experience as psychologist, teacher, and above all, good friend to the deaf community echoes through this volume. Although five of seven chapters were authored by me, they were carefully reviewed by Dr. Vernon, who added the sensitive points that only experience and deep commitment make possible.

As our discussions developed, they ranged from the considerations of the individual child, to the nature of the professional and lay communities which have allowed a perpetuation of mythical notions as to "what is good for the deaf child." In the writing, there was a progressive broadening of the perspective; although knowledge gained from each of the individual areas which we examined seemed to hold promise for giving "the answer" to the resistance to needed changes, we were still left feeling that the "complete answer" had not been found. This feeling remained until we came to understand that answers to questions about deaf children can only be found in examining the whole of their life circumstances as an integrated process.

With the completion of the book, we are left with the unsettled feeling that understanding of the deaf community by the hearing community is limited. In our search, we have learned much about the hearing community, not only how it has dealt with deaf people by denying their unique needs and suppressing their difference, but how society at large tends to maintain itself by carefully controlling various groups that tend to disrupt its equilibrium. Deaf persons have been overcontrolled; the threat that deaf persons will be disruptive because of their differences is more imagined than real.

Perhaps many times as one reads this book, he will ask "Of what relevance is this or that issue?" What is contained here represents the authors' ideas of what issues are relevant. The relevance cannot always be explicitly documented; to do so, in each instance, would require many additional volumes. Our hoped-for result is that enough areas will seem relevant to enough people so that they can then develop the meaningfulness more than in the present effort.

Our traditional approach to understanding deaf people has been to look at areas in which they have failed, then to reasons for those failures. Originally, explanations centered around the idea that failures, especially educational failures, were intrinsically related to deafness. A series of psychological studies were published in support of that premise. Some still regard deaf children as intrinsically retarded and admonish parents to expect no more than fifth-grade academic achievement. Dr. Vernon has been one of the leaders in defeating this destructive idea through research, articles, and speeches. The deaf child's intelligence had originally been examined by using standard verbal intelligence tests. The baseline for comparison was the scores of hearing children. That the deaf child has a major sensory deficit precludes the use of such materials without careful and considered modification.

We are writing as psychiatrist and psychologist, but psychiatric and psychological aspects of deafness are only a part of the total problem. Paradoxically, despite their significance, they have probably received the least objective, scientific attention. There have been a few books covering these psychiatric and psychological phenomena, but when all of the categories of published material on deafness are compared for sheer volume, psychological works constitute only a small portion. Neither normative language development nor normative psychological development can be taken for granted in the deaf child. Normal patterns of language or psychological development do not adequately serve as baselines for behavior in the deaf child. One hope is that this book will help to clarify distinctions in linguistic and psychological development of deaf children.

Another hoped-for result of this effort is overcoming one of the chief obstacles to progressive development of services for deaf children. This is the failure to develop effective interactions and coalitions between parents and professionals. Parents of young deaf children seldom know or speak to the parents of older deaf children or to deaf adults. Communication between these groups is vital to the growth of a parent's understanding of deaf children. We want to help parents and professionals concerned with the deaf child to see the whole of the problem, not just bits and pieces related to this or that aspect of the problem; i.e., to see themselves and deaf children "in perspective."

One of the main complaints of deaf children and adults is the isolation they feel from their families and community. Such complaints are not less frequent from deaf people educated in traditional oral programs. We shall demonstrate why the many hours spent acquiring an oral technique do not necessarily establish feelings of closeness between human beings. Closeness comes from meaningful exchanges of information and feeling; in short, from understanding and empathy.

One of man's greatest assets is also one of his greatest liabilities: the capacity to probe and learn. We are made to learn, to grow, and to change. When this does not occur, we suffer. Just as our muscles become flabby and inefficient when we lie ill in bed, so our minds lie fallow when they are not allowed to function as they were intended.

The thought of being isolated from one's fellow human beings and from the sound environment in which we live is painful for all to contemplate. If we did not have to be isolated, if we could understand what the intentions of the other persons were, if we could explore the richness of their behavior, if we could delve into the world's literature, then the loss of hearing would not be so intense. But without adequate language, we cannot do these things. This is why deaf persons are isolated.

They grow in silence, but they need not grow alone. For centuries, the deaf have been one of nature's "experiments" on the effects of cultural isolation. But for all its years, this "experiment" has resulted in little to bring the deaf into the mainstream as equals. When all of the academic and pseudo-academic rhetoric generated over how best to educate and socialize the deaf is over, they and they alone must live out the "results." The results, when examined honestly, are not encouraging. But by early appropriate intervention at the social and educational level today and tomorrow, the deaf child and his family need not continue to be strangers in the same house.

Contributing Authors

Valerie Feldman, M.Ed., J.D.
Formerly Child Development Specialist, Siegel Institute, Michael Reese Hospital and Medical Center, Chicago.

Bonnie Litowitz, Ph.D.
Associate Professor, Northwestern University, Department of Linguistics and Department of Communicative Sciences, Evanston.

Noel Matkin, Ph.D.,
Professor, Department of Speech & Hearing Science, University of Arizona, Tucson.

Rachael Mayberry, Ph.D.
Research Associate (Assistant Professor), Department of Education, University of Chicago, Chicago.

Eugene D. Mindel, M.D.
Chairman, Mental Health Department, PruCare of Illinois; Senior Psychiatric Consultant, Mental Health Services for Deaf Adults and Children, Siegel Institute, Michael Reese Hospital and Medical Center, Chicago.

Barbara Rayson, M.A.
Clinical Psychologist, Siegel Institute, Michael Reese Hospital and Medical Center, Chicago.

Laszlo Stein, Ph.D.
Director, Siegel Institute, Michael Reese Hospital and Medical Center and, Associate Professor Department of Surgery (Otolaryngology) University of Chicago, Chicago.

McCay Vernon, Ph.D.
Professor of Psychology, Western Maryland College, Westminster.

Rhonda Wodlinger-Cohen, M.A.
Research Assistant, Department of Education, University of Chicago, Chicago.

CHAPTER 1

The Impact of Deaf Children on Their Families

Eugene D. Mindel
Valerie Feldman

T his chapter focuses on the development of deaf children and their families from the time when parents' suspicions of a disability first develop, through their confrontation with the definitive diagnosis of deafness, and beyond, through the difficult and often painful adjustments that must be made to the disability. The purpose of this book is to give readers greater insight into the emotional frustrations that deaf children and their parents experience. These insights will translate into enhanced empathy toward affected families, ultimately leading to stronger communication through emotional, cognitive, and linguistic growth.

Traditionally, services offered to deaf children and their families have been within the confines of a number of nonintegrated parochial frameworks. Services generally have included audiology, education, speech training and lip-reading, social work, psychology, and psychiatry. The professionals offering these services often work independently of each other; needed services can be duplicated or overlooked. For example, most educational programs for deaf children do not adequately provide for the emotional needs of parents, which are ordinarily considered the province of the psychosocial disciplines. Parents locked into unresolved depressions as a consequence of bearing deaf children are less available emotionally to their children and can negatively affect their children's educational progress.

The following discussion attempts to give parents and professionals a full and accurate perspective on the total social and psychological system in which they participate in the early years of deaf childrens' lives. Failure to acknowledge all parts of the family and community systems that deaf children enter does not eliminate the importance of any unacknowledged parts of the total system; these will surface regardless. If their influence is not acknowledged, they can act as obstacles to successful total rehabilitation. For example, the failure by professionals to consider the need for early distinct and clear communication between parents and children may restrict the ultimate educational and emotional development of deaf children.

The parents' discovery of their child's deafness happens not in an instant of stunning revelation; they may feel that it does, however, because of their intense emotional reactions to a professional saying, "Your child is deaf." In truth, this painful moment verifies a gradual accumulation of observations suggesting that the child's development is not normal. How readily parents respond to these clues depends upon a variety of influences addressed in this chapter, including the parents' personalities; the state of their marriage during the conception, gestation, birth, and early years of life of their child; the parents' relationships to their own parents; whether or not the deaf child is their first child; and the knowledge and sensitivity of members of the professional community who are consulted.

PARENTS' PERSONALITIES

Various traits of the parents' personalities significantly influence their initial awareness or lack of awareness of their child's deafness. During the child's early months, only subtle behaviors suggest the presence of deafness. The discovery may be delayed by an unusual amount of denial, rationalization, and procrastination beyond the time when subtle behaviors become obvious (e.g., seemingly variable responses to the parents' voices become more predictable). Similarly, later parental decisions requiring shifts in emphasis or orientation may occur slowly and after the optimal time. (Examples of such decisions are when to request psychiatric help for children showing emotional problems and when to provide for special education of children who are discovered to have learning disabilities in addition to deafness).

Personality is described here in terms of adaptive capacities that define a person's ability to cope with unanticipated occurrences. By studying the various ways that people respond to novel and unusual situations at different points in the process of their growth and maturity, their capacity to adapt to life generally can be assessed.

Consideration of the parents' capacities to cope with a deaf child is appropriate at this point. An examination of each parent's response to greater-than-average stress sheds light on the subject: How did the parent deal with the social and sexual challenges of early adolescence (demonstrating effectiveness of response to maturational challenges)? Is there a history of juvenile delinquency (demonstrating limited ability to delay gratification)? Is there a spotty employment record (demonstrating inability to persevere)?

During gestation, the mother psychologically relates to the fetus as if it were part of her own body. She projects onto it fears, expectations, and other emotions derived from her own childhood. Many of the mother's thoughts during pregnancy are directed toward the nurturing environment that she proposes to provide for the child; such thoughts are especially common with the first child. There is hopefulness for the child's future. Parents from troubled homes often take an optimistic vow: "With my child, it will be different." Feelings related to the current marital situation can also influence the way in which the mother relates to her child. In an unhappy marriage, anger can be displaced from the mother onto the unborn child rather than directly onto the husband.

If the newborn shows no obvious physical abnormalities at birth, the infant and mother enter into a relationship in which the mother's expectations and feelings for the infant blend with the infant's personality. The infants' initial repertory of actions is primarily instinctual and not greatly different from that of other infants, and the mother's reactions and interpretations of her child's behavior are based on aspects of her own personality projected onto the child. However, infants do differ in their evident endowment at birth. Some are placid and easily cared for; others are irritable and difficult to please. The manner in which the mother deals with an uncomfortable infant is one measure of her ability to cope with her own frustrations. The newborn infant crying in hunger, pain, or fatigue can trigger strong emotions such as rage, which may derive in part from difficulty in determining easily the sources of the child's discomfort. With a deaf child, this issue continues long beyond the period of infancy. Thus, the deaf child must develop adequate methods to communicate important feelings at an early age.

Deafness often is not diagnosed until many months after it is first suspected. In many cases, parents' suspicions are discounted by a physician on the assumption that the baby "will outgrow it." The mother–infant relationship can be jeopardized during these months by the inability of each to pick up on and make meaning of the other's vocalizations. This subtle breach in communication confounds and delays the diagnosis of deafness.

As one mother described her experiences during the months prior to the diagnosis of her son's deafness, "I thought it was me. I thought that I was just a bad mother." The feeling reflected in this statement is repeatedly expressed, both verbally and nonverbally, by mothers who were not consciously aware of their children's deafness in the earliest months.

> A major factor contributing to (parental) anxiety is the lack of . . . gratification. Deafness is an invisible handicap where unease remains ill-defined because the real handicap of the deaf child is unclear. The child may not turn and smile on hearing the parents' voice. Such behavior may be seen as negative rather than based on a physical deficit. Parents need to feel love from their children. A child who gives little response often leaves the parent feeling empty. I have experienced, as have many of the parents I have worked with, the feeling of being a "bad" parent or of being a little crazy for not being able to define what was wrong with my child and with my parenting. I was caught in the isolation of an undefined stress.[1]

In the mother's role as a provider and as a buffer between infant and surroundings, she finds that certain of the child's approaches and assaults on the environment are acceptable, and others not. For example, some mothers enjoy a small boy's aggression; they view it as harmless. As the toddler moves about the home, occasionally damaging prized possessions, they accept this behavior. Other mothers are antagonized by such aggression and readily punish the child.

Similarly, a child's affectionate advances are placed on a scale of values; a child's affection can be regarded as "too much" or "not enough." The mother's attitudes are of particular importance during the infant's first year of life because of her close and constant contact with the infant. The father may rarely be home when the baby is awake. Later, the child's personality development also comes under the influence of father as well as members of the extended family; yet the mother's personality generally has the greatest influence on the child.

Deaf children, because they are denied access to verbal communication, remain more dependent on their mothers than do normally hearing children. This dependence is born of an inability to develop conventional communication, which forces them to use the actions, not the words of the few people with whom they are familiar. Strangers, as a rule, do not provide a good learning opportunity for deaf children. Only rarely can strangers easily handle the difficulties inherent in such social interactions with deaf children as spontaneous communication and play.

Because of the severely restricted choice of people from whom to learn, what the mother regards as acceptable and unacceptable is firmly implanted on the deaf child's personality.

> The absence of speech skills makes deafness "visible" (or rather, audible), and emphasizes the differences between parents and child. These are some of the emotional reasons for the tremendous emphasis placed on the learning of oral skills. . . . But the unwillingness of hearing parents and teachers to accept a second, different communicative mode is often so strong as to reflect feelings of stigma regarding differences.[2]

The deaf child's forced dependence upon the mother imposes additional frustrations on her. She cannot extricate herself physically or emotionally from the care of the child through outside activities. Even a working mother, who has provided for her child's normal daytime activities through school or babysitting arrangements, must forgo a day's employment when the child becomes ill or needs special examination. The child's needs are primary. Some mothers view this situation as burdensome and intolerable.

Economic and financial circumstances frequently demand that a mother, whether single or married, earn income to sustain an acceptable standard of living. The number of working mothers has increased sharply the past decade. Feelings of guilt and sadness aroused in women who have given birth to deaf children may be exacerbated when they delegate care of the child to others so they can go to work. For instance, where does the mother find a baby-sitter competent in the use of sign language? Baby-sitters or day-care programs will only rarely accept handicapped children. Rare also is the employer who agrees to release a mother once or twice a week to attend a parent-infant program; often, the mother is forced to reduce her working hours or terminate her job in order to remain at home with the child. In either case, the mother's emotional and financial stress under these conditions is compounded by feelings of helplessness and despair in the earliest stages after the diagnosis of deafness is established.

Any efforts made by a parent–child program to take into consideration the child's alternative caretakers or the parent's employers can serve well all involved parties. For example, a personal phone call or letter to an employer may yield a sympathetic response. Subsequently, the employer becomes educated about deafness and the needs of the employee's family. Parents may receive time off because of efforts made by professionals to incorporate the employers in an extended caretaking network.

In most family systems, the daytime work activities of the deaf child's father remain unaltered, but his evening and weekend family hours are altered. Demands are made on his emotional resources to cope with his family's redirection to an orbit now centered around a child with special demands.

Whereas the mother derives considerable emotional compensation from the physical nurturance and nonverbal communication with the deaf child, the father may begin to feel like a satellite being. Almost nothing in his background has equipped him to adapt readily to the special nature of fathering a deaf child. Unsuccessful coping can produce changes in the father's personality. The father of a handicapped child may suffer from diminished self-esteem in addition to greater marital dissatisfaction.

Many males react to the special nurturing needs of a deaf child as an assault on their masculinity. The deaf child, forced into greater dependence upon the parents, is seen as unnaturally passive, especially if that child is a male. Using the hands for communicating may seem strangely unmanly. Far fewer fathers than mothers become competent signers, due in part to the fact that many sign language instruction programs are offered only during daytime working hours.

INFLUENCE OF THE FAMILY
ENVIRONMENT

Although the parents' personalities are important in relation to the deaf child, so too are the collective personality factors of the marriage relationship. A marriage is a human system initially comprised of two separate persons. Eventually it assumes and contains characteristics resulting from the interactions of the two personalities and the acquired memories of their shared life experiences.

The relationships a couple have had with their parents exert considerable influence on their own marriage. What parents experienced as children in their own homes creates the expectations and patterns of behavior in their marriage. Separations and divorces often occur in families in which similar occurrences took place in the previous generation, and frequently for the same reasons. Punitive child-rearing practices are commonly passed down through offspring. If these conflicts are severe and nonadaptive, greater disturbance can occur in the offspring than was evident in the parents or grandparents.

A. B., a 35-year-old mother of three children, had a history of recurrent depressions. Her 11-year-old daughter had been in a residential treatment center for more than one year and was diagnosed as having childhood schizophrenia. A. B. had had a poor relationship with her own mother, an egocentric, demanding, and often cold woman. Her father usually put drinking at the local tavern ahead of his family responsibilities. The daughter was born a few months after the death of A. B.'s mother, and her birth reactivated A. B.'s conflicts, leaving her depressed and unavailable — her emotional investment still belonged to her own mother. During her daughter's earliest years, A. B. and her daughter replayed A. B.'s relationship with her own cold and hostile mother.

In assessing the capacity of a couple to cope with the stresses that evolve in the course of marriage, the concern of this text is the reaction to the stress of having a child who is noncommunicative or who will never communicate in a conventional way. The following background information may be helpful.

Each parent has built-in expectations for his or her child. As a child develops the ability to communicate, the parent generally transmits these expectations through speech, although some expectations are communicated nonverbally. The child analyzes the environment and learns the "house rules." Some rules are interpreted by parents more liberally than others. Absolute "must nots" may be emphasized by physical punishment. Lesser prohibitions may be treated more leniently. This apparent ambiguity can lead to confusion for the deaf child. *Ambiguity in communication is one of the deaf child's greatest problems in the home.* This is especially true during the "terrible twos," when a child tests the limits of the parents' coping abilities. Even for families who are fluent in total communication (simultaneous speaking and signing), the messages often appear mixed. Parents may feel ambivalent toward the child, wanting to treat him or her as "normal," yet not wanting to deny wants or wishes. The deaf child frequently senses this ambivalence, particularly when the expression on the parent's face does not match the message on the parent's hands. Even with total communication, the mother generally is the primary facilitator of communication between the deaf child and other family members. Conversation from father must go through mother to be interpreted rather than directly to the child. Under these circumstances, misunderstandings, misconceptions, and mixed messages abound.

For deaf children even more than for hearing children, inconsistent limits cause perplexity and confusion. If this happens often, deaf children tend to further restrict their activities to avoid stressful states of confusion and anxiety. They may limit activities to those known to be safe and predictably acceptable to the parents. Their emotional and social growth become restricted.

Parents ideally should function as a consistent unit in the formation of house rules. When they establish rules independent of each other, further confusion is added to the deaf child's environment. Ambiguity can occur because many attitudes in the marriage develop nonverbally. By mere observation, a husband or wife may intuit the partner's attitude toward the deaf child's behavior. It is impossible for parents to discuss explicitly the full range of their attitudes about the child's various activities. Often, only those actions of the child that stimulate conflict in the parents are discussed between them; many times even these are not discussed. The parents' capacity to negotiate their disagreements over expectations and ideals determines how successful they are in managing the difficult situations that arise in the raising of their deaf child.

At 2½ years, Johnny regularly attended a parent-infant program with his mother, a full-time homemaker. His father, Mr. R., was a factory laborer who frequently worked overtime. When he arrived home each evening, Mr. R. would roughhouse with Johnny. This play was both stimulating and exciting for his son. Their formal communication was limited to gestures and a few formal signs. By dinnertime, Mr. R. was ready to have a quiet evening meal. Unable to communicate his wish to Johnny, Mr. R. would request that Mrs. R. take the responsibility of calming Johnny. But Johnny delighted in the father-son play and had no intention to calm down. Mother became the ogre as she tried to convey father's wishes to Johnny. The latter, a keen observer of his environment, learned quickly how to make everyone excited and disagreeable. Johnny would throw daily tantrums in order to coerce his parents into responding to his wishes. His tantrums became a tactic to test his parents' ability to make decisions for him. Only when Mr. and Mrs. R. began to respond consistently and without ambiguity did Johnny begin to understand the limits and expectations placed on him.

Rarely is either parent experienced in rearing a deaf youngster; nor do they know other parents of deaf children. They often agonize in ignorance or with misinformation over their decisions for appropriate action. As a result, they may displace their frustrated feelings onto each other. Those marital conflicts that cannot be solved successfully affect the entire marriage. Parents may be thwarted in achieving anticipated parental and marital gratification. However, when they can mutually redirect their expectations and appreciate their deaf child's conforming to real rather than imagined capacities, they achieve much satisfaction.

The single mother presents a special situation. She does not have those support systems that are available in a stable marriage. The sharing of ideas, thoughts, and feelings around raising a handicapped child may be limited to extended family members or to friends who are not living with the deaf child on a daily basis, and who thereby do not necessarily understand the joys and frustrations the single mother faces.

WHEN THE DEAF CHILD IS THE FIRST CHILD

A significant factor influencing the time of discovery of a child's deafness is position in the sibship. With a first child, the mother does not know what behaviors to expect as indicators that a child is hearing. With later children, the now more sensitive and observing mother has drawn up a mental schedule of expected growth and development. Thus, the experienced parent often suspects deafness sooner in the child who does not respond to the mother's voice at 3 months by cooing, who does not search for voices at 4 months, who is not calmed by sound, or whose first words do not occur on schedule.

INFLUENCE OF THE EXTENDED FAMILY

The nature of the parent-grandparent ties exerts considerable influence on the raising of the deaf child. In some cases, the deaf child and mother live in the same household with the grandmother. The grandmother may, in fact, be the child's primary caretaker if the mother works or goes to school.

From their own fathers and mothers the deaf child's parents have derived ideals about parenthood as well as about social and professional achievement. These ideals are deeply embedded and automatically influence behavior. Parents first discovering deafness may see themselves as failing to achieve a desired goal for their child. When parents perceive their failure to achieve a desired goal, their disappointment and concern threads back to the ever-present question, "What will mother and father think?" If the deaf child's parents sense failure, doubts and worries develop. In contrast, if they realize that they have lived up to the standards consonant with their ideals, as largely influenced by their own parents, a feeling of success and optimism prevails.

In typical relationships between a deaf child's parents and grandparents, such concerns and attitudes flow naturally. If parents with strong ties to their own parents have a relationship that functions as parent-child rather than adult-adult, their interactions may be more stressful than gratifying. In such a relationship, the deaf child's parents still look to their parents for reassurance and confirmation as they grow in their own parenting roles. A feeling that they have failed to receive such reassurance creates pervasive and possibly enduring anger between the generations.

In some families, the grandparents may not want to interfere or may believe that they do not know how to raise a deaf child. They may prefer not to baby-sit or provide other supportive services to the young parents due to their feelings of discomfort, ambivalence, or guilt. Where parents and grandparents reach an agreement as to their proper roles, the relationship tends to be warm and comfortable. There is mutual recognition and respect.

The parents can turn to the grandparents for guidance when there is feeling that the latters' experience will contribute to the direction of their own lives.

Fifteen-month-old Joshua attended a parent-infant program regularly with his mother and father. Because there was no program within the local community, Mr. and Mrs. T drove 1 1/2 hours each way to attend. Either Joshua's maternal or paternal grandmother accompanied them; frequently his grandfather or aunts attended as well. Family members were invited to participate in the playroom or to observe through one-way observation mirror. The involvement of the extended family had a positive effect. Each family member was able to ask his or her own questions: "What is the sign for fire engine?" "Is there an operation to correct Joshua's hearing loss?" In addition, each was able to directly contribute to the sessions, speaking about Joshua from his or her own perspective. "When Joshua is at my house, he loves to climb the stairs." "He does not respond to the sound of the tractor on our farm." The family's questions and contributions were sensitive and thoughtful, and added to a supportive environment for all who participated.

Frequently grandparents or well-meaning friends reinforce the parents' own wishful thinking with such statements as "He's just stubborn — all 2-year-olds are like that." "You didn't talk until you were almost 3. He's just like you." "He's not talking because he has an older brother who says everything for him." In other words, parents are being told that what they see and think to be true is probably not true. This ill-conceived effort shields parents from their feelings about having a deaf child. The grandparents also try to shield themselves from the feelings provoked by the deafness. The grandchild is seen as an extension of their own child, and hence an extension of themselves. Thus, the psychological problems do not affect family members in isolation. Because of the interplay of feelings in the family unit, all members are affected in various ways.

The responsibilities that fall particularly to the mother of the newly diagnosed deaf child may be overwhelming. She generally is the one person who attends parent-infant programs on a regular basis. She alone must receive information, understand the curriculum and teaching methods, maintain the hearing aid, learn sign language, and so on. At home she must explain this information to father, to the grandparents, to friends, and to neighbors. They may proceed to ask questions that she, in turn, must bring back to the program the following week. The inclusion of extended family members, as well as neighbors and friends, in the education of the child can be crucial. If others are unable to attend the program, support can be provided by sending home materials, by phone conversations, and by special "family days" in the evenings or on weekends.

Trisha was a mature, vibrant 3-year-old who had contracted meningitis at the age of 2½ and who was referred for short-term placement in a parent-infant program prior to fall admission to a preschool class. Sandra, her unmarried mother, was mature and patient. Mother and daughter had moved from Sandra's mother's home into their own home across the street, spurred by Sandra's differences with her own mother over raising Trisha, especially after she became deaf. Trisha and Sandra shopped, ate, and played together. Although initially, Trisha's emotional, physical, and cognitive needs were seemingly well met, it soon became apparent that Sandra's needs were not being met. While she was giving much of herself to her young daughter, the impact of Trisha's hearing loss became more than Sandra could bear. Sandra did not want to return to the confines of her mother's home; she nonetheless wanted her mother's emotional nurturance. Sandra's mother attended several of the parent-infant sessions. She initially remained aloof, perhaps to protect herself from the pain of losing both daughter and granddaughter. Over ensuing weeks the vibrancy and playfulness of both Trisha and Sandra lessened. A counselor began to help Sandra verbalize her sorrow, particularly emphasizing Sandra's ambivalence over separation from her mother. Within a short period of time, Sandra recognized that she needed her mother for many reasons. Sandra soon invited her mother to join her in discussions with the counselor. Desirous of uniting once again with her daughter and granddaughter, Sandra's mother agreed. In the end, Sandra chose to maintain her own apartment and her independence. As a result of the discussions, Sandra's mother could better understand Sandra's needs and feelings. She could begin again to give emotional support and guidance. This in turn had salutary effects on Sandra and Trisha's mother-child relationship.

PSYCHOLOGICAL RESPONSES TO
DISCOVERY OF DEAFNESS

When parents are confronted with the realization that their child is not responding to sounds, various psychological responses occur. These tend to prevent parents from becoming aware of things that cause them psychic pain. Parents experience blends of emotion interfering with their sense of well-being. Concerns lurk in the background and modify the typical emotional climate of the home, in which a child's spontaneity and innocence usually create an air of hopefulness and pleasure. The dim awareness of their child's hearing loss has cast a shadow of doubt.

Dynamic psychiatry has identified a number of mechanisms by which human beings cope with stressful and unexpected occurrences. Many of these mechanisms are classified as adaptive behaviors — the capacity of a person to cope with the unanticipated. The more unique, complex, and stressful the occurrence, the more it taxes one's capacity for adaptive behavior.

When the evidence that a child is not hearing becomes rationally incontrovertible, a parent experiences psychic pain. In thinking about this, the parent may only allow himself or herself to recognize the nature of what is perceived in such a way to obscure the true picture. Thus, the question of a child's hearing loss still may remain unanswered.

Denial and Rationalization

Two of the known psychological mechanisms by which reality is partially obscured are *denial* and *rationalization*. Parents may be able to perceive the real nature of a situation. However, in interpreting their perceptions, parents may exclude certain essential elements that would give an accurate assessment of the child's hearing capacity. As intellect leads inexorably toward painful realizations, feelings, stimulated by anticipated psychic pain, cause an abandonment or alteration in the nature of certain important perceptions, so that understanding remains incomplete. The initial reaction to emotional shock is disbelief. Disbelief eventually formalizes into denial.

Feelings can blur perception through a psychological denial that disregards certain elements of the child's total behavior. For example, parents may ignore the child's failure to respond to voices. They notice the child shift gaze toward a door that has just been closed, and attribute this to a perception of sound rather than to the strong vibrations transmitted through the floor or the blocking of incoming light. The child may creep or crawl toward a television or stereo, putting an ear close to it. With residual hearing, the child may even be alerted to loud environmental sounds such as the roar of a low-flying jet, the loud ringing of a doorbell, or the sharp bang of a slammed screen door. However, this does not mean that the child can perceive the crucial and more complex sound patterns of the human voice. In these examples, the parents deny the hearing loss through misinterpreting the significance of a response to light, vibrations, or crude noises.

Another psychological operation relevant to our discussion is rationalization. Rationalization creates fictionalized alternatives that replace the more realistic and pain-inducing explanations of the facts observed. Some rationalizations are culturally determined. Deafness may not be seen immediately as the reason for the child's lack of responsiveness to sound. Instead, the youngster is described as "just being stubborn" or "hearing what he wants to hear." Other reasons may be invoked, such as a family history of "late talkers."

Where lack of hearing is the plausible explanation, the parent, as illustrated above, may use other factors concurrent in the environment to create an explanation other than deafness for the child's failure to hear. This is the essence of rationalization.

> Tony entered a parent-infant program at 3 years of age, after he was diagnosed as a profoundly deaf child. His mother, Mrs. H. explained that, while she knew Tony was not responsive at 12 months as her other children had been, she thought "he was just stubborn." He did say "mama" and "baba" (for bottle). By 18 months, Tony had little formal expressive language and did not respond to others talking to him. Mrs. H. thought "he was just slow" since "boys are usually slower than girls at talking." When Tony was 2 years old, Mrs. H. began to question whether something was wrong. She was assured when the doctor told her, "He's a happy, healthy baby; he'll start talking soon." There were other late talkers in her family. By the time Tony was 2 1/2, Mrs. H. thought perhaps he was retarded. She took him to a local preschool screening center. Tony performed well on nonver-

bal tests but fell far behind on speech and language items that required auditory and verbal abilities. He then was referred for an audiological evaluation, at which time his hearing loss was diagnosed.

Definitive diagnosis of the hearing loss sensitively rendered will interrupt denial and rationalization. With the rendering of the diagnosis, the parents' fears that their child cannot hear are presumptively confirmed, and they will experience what most parents call *shock.*

Shock

Regardless of the child's age, a period of shock follows the parents' learning that their child is deaf. The shock is a blend of disbelief and grief, helplessness, anger, and guilt. A person thrust into such a state suddenly feels set apart from others, who seem happier, content, not burdened with grief, scarcely if at all noticing their pain.

The disbelief the parents feel is a continuation of the earlier period of doubt. Gradually, as the acute grieving abates, the utter disbelief is supplanted by the question, "Why did it happen to me?" Some parents consciously regard the child's deafness as punishment for imagined past transgressions; others feel it simply as punishment but are unable to perceive reasons. Some mothers recall having had fantasies during pregnancy of bearing a damaged child.

All expectant mothers have ambivalent feelings toward the growing fetus. Its birth and subsequent development promise gratification. However, prior to birth the fetus derives unremittingly its share of nourishment and contributes increasingly to physical discomfort. Under stress, after discovering the child's disability, a mother may recall angry fantasies about the unborn child and mixed feelings about parenthood. She may associate these past feelings causally with the child's handicap and thereby feel responsible for the deafness. Intense feelings of guilt may ensue.

The dynamics and development of these feelings require explanations. Anger is a natural consequence of frustration and disappointment. Like all emotions, it seeks an object. Because of being disabled, the child may become the object toward whom anger is directed. Although parents consciously realize the child had no choice in his or her destiny, they may, nonetheless, discover negative feelings toward the child. This in turn stimulates further guilt.

Parents must know, when possible, the cause of the child's deafness, whatever the cause might be. Knowing the cause, and with psychological support, they can begin to realistically face issues about which they would otherwise fantasize. "Why didn't you tell me you had a deaf uncle?" "The doctor never told me rubella could cause deafness." "I shouldn't have worked with young children while I was pregnant." "How will this syndrome affect our children and our children's children?"

Anger originates from partial loss of maternal gratification early in the deaf child's life. The mother's gratification normally arises from observing her baby's contentment after feedings or caring for other physical needs. It increases in observing the child's attainment of growth and developmental milestones. If these satisfactions do not occur or are diminished, the mother feels hurt and inadequate. If they are attained, they confirm her success. The disabled child leaves the mother feeling partially fulfilled or unfulfilled as she looks for those accomplishments that are the rewards of her investment of time and love.

Anger also stems from the helplessness and confusion of not having anticipated a deaf child's birth. The parents know little of what to expect or what to do. As they gradually realize the limitations imposed by deafness, they feel helpless because they cannot change it. As the child moves into the formative years for speech and language, parents feel helpless in communicating basic information and conveying fundamental needs. They feel even more helpless when the child is fretting and can communicate only as much as squeals, grunts, tears, and gestures will convey.

The mother experiences frustration trying to cope with a child whom she cannot understand and who cannot understand her. Moreover, she feels helpless in attempting to express her feelings sufficiently to gain relief from this seemingly unresolvable dilemma. Inevitably, those things seen as interfering with basic capacities to cope with the environment are likely to cause a sense of inadequacy. This too can stimulate anger. Thus, the presence of the deaf child in the family often causes unremitting frustration and anger. The casual observer is unaware of why this is happening.

Considerable support is provided parents of newly diagnosed deaf children by meeting and talking with other parents who have been through a similar experience. The sharing of joys as well as frustrations helps the parents to see that the deafness does in fact have an impact on the family, yet joys exist as well. Parents must eventually view their children as "communicative beings" with their own thoughts, feelings, and ideas. Often, only after the child uses his or her first formal sign do parents clearly realize that the child is not retarded.

EMPATHY AND OVERIDENTIFICATION

We tend to view other people through our own frames of reference. Thoughts and feelings about various people and situations that we impute to others are often projections of our own personalities. These egocentric reactions color our perceptions of the life circumstances of others. If accurate, our perceptions are said to show *empathy*. With our children, empathy is the most intense.

The child's development is influenced by the manner in which parents' thoughts and feelings contribute to the psychological structure of the home. Parents who only partially understand the true nature of the child's deafness may *overidentify* with his or her position: On viewing their child's situation subjectively, certain aspects will seem more stressful to them than they actually are to the child. This represents an overidentification with the child. It is an inaccurate, exaggerated conception of the situation. The parents are seeing the deaf child more through their own frames of reference than the child's. Empathy implies a realistic appraisal of the disability. Overidentification is a pathological extension of empathy.

Those things that tend to interfere with basic capacities when coping with parent-child interactions are likely to stimulate anger in the child and the parents. The source of the parents' anger often is their overidentification. They have projected for themselves a concept of being a deaf child. This emphasizes the aspects of deafness that seem important to them because of their psychological needs. In contrast, the deaf child's anger may have a different source, stemming from those situations when he or she wants to communicate and cannot.

A mother tends to perceive her child as an extension of herself. This is especially prominent in the earliest phases of the child's life. Even though the child has only the rudiments of an adult personality, the mother tends to impute motivations that are in fact her own projections. Some of her pleasure comes in thinking how it would feel to be taken care of in the way that she is caring for the child. Things that she perceives as hurtful or helpful, hating or loving to her will be interpreted likewise for the child. If a part of the child is defective, the mother will think about this as she imagines she would experience it herself. When doing this, she interprets her child's state as if she were suddenly deprived of the capacity to hear. Various fantasies related to the importance of hearing and the associated unconscious psychological conflicts are projected as being the child's feelings. These projections may not be at all identical with the child's real feelings.

There are, then, two aspects of deafness with which parents can empathize or overidentify. The first is the loss of hearing itself. Consciously and intellectually parents understand that the loss means not being able to get information through hearing. Unconsciously, they may experience this loss as a form of bodily injury. The second aspect is the social isolation consequent to deafness.

Deafness Perceived as Bodily Injury

Various attitudes develop toward bodily injury. Universally, people regard the loss of any body part as a diminution of security.[3] We feel less secure because there is less equipment with which to adapt to stressful situations or enjoy pleasure-yielding opportunities. Some losses that are physically small are psychologically large. A study of 19 mothers of children having congenital heart disease demonstrated that the psychological effect was not so much dependent upon the severity of the defect as it was upon how the mother perceived it. The longer a mother lived with her child, the more prone to distortion became her perception of the defect.[4]

In part, the significance of a loss depends upon the age it is incurred. Children with early limb amputations do not experience the self-consciousness and awkwardness such losses produce later in life when the body part is not only an integral part of the person's function in the physical sense, but has become invested with a variety of psychological meanings. People having losses at a later age give up not only part of themselves, but must also alter psychological representations that have become a complete part of their self-concept and internalized body image.

Deafness is a far more complicated process than the loss of a body part. The child deaf from birth does not experience deafness as a loss in the sense of having had hearing. The parents, however, because of their empathic relationship, experience the child's congenital deafness as a loss. From the outset, the congenital hearing loss alters the nature of the child's contact with the world. Information normally obtained through the modality of hearing is not available, leading to profound influences on subsequent psychological and social development. As deaf children between the ages of 2 and 5 become cognitively aware of differences between themselves and others and come to understand that there is such a thing as hearing, they begin the work of adjusting themselves to life in a hearing world.

Deafness and Social Isolation

The second factor that parents consider within the context of an empathic relationship with their deaf child is the isolation imposed by deafness. The extent of this isolation is a matter of degree. With profound hearing loss, children will be virtually excluded from information and human contact ordinarily available through hearing. This means the loss of that early parent-infant relationship conveyed through sound. During those early rudimentary communications between a parent and infant, the baby coos in response to the parent's voice. The human voice is a vehicle for feeling, and parent vocalization during the caretaking process is one way of communicating feelings. Deafness isolates children from these feelings in their parents' voices.

A more profound progressive isolation from the hearing world begins at the point when children begin to depend upon auditory stimulation for the development of language and general knowledge. Residual hearing insufficient to allow children to understand speech isolates them from conventional language usage. However, remnants of hearing serve to alert children to the presence of other people and to loud environmental sounds. Hard-of-hearing children may or may not have a richer language development than totally deaf children. Nevertheless, they experience some sense of isolation in situations where they cannot be full participants in conversation. This is especially true in group interactions or in areas filled with prominent background noises.

Though this book is concerned primarily with profoundly deaf children, we should mention that all too often parents and educators have the unrealistic expectation that hard-of-hearing children can be fully integrated into the hearing world. Closer examination of the social and psychological situation of these children and adults reveals that they are acutely sensitive to their differences and to the lack of understanding of their difficulties by well-meaning hearing people.[5] This is especially true when they are placed in situations requiring that they conform to classroom and social activities geared to those who have no hearing loss. Significant gaps in knowledge have been demonstrated where the lack of hearing results in the failure to understand classroom instruction. The written language of congenitally hard-of-hearing children generally reveals what they have missed.

As deaf children mature and recognize that oral conversation and reading are the chief modes of communication and learning, their sense of isolation increases. Without benefit of total communication, they must still resort to action and gesture to communicate wishes. Should parents demand speech and lipreading as the only acceptable form of communication, feelings of isolation will be intensified and cognitive deprivation increased.[6]

The parents' feelings, crystallizing around their concept of hearing loss as a bodily injury, represent a distinctly different psychological orientation toward deafness from that of the deaf child. Ordinarily they do not reconcile this difference. The psychological distinction between growing up deaf and growing up hearing is profound. A central thesis to this work is that the degree of isolation is an area open for correction through total communication.

Uninvited isolation from others is one of the most painful of human sufferings. No one can survive in a vacuum. Our capacity to communicate meaningfully with others is inextricably tied to our capacity for living. Diminished communication renders one compromised. Nonexistent communication renders one impotent.

The grief, anger, guilt, and helplessness stimulated by the discovery of the child's deafness seldom disappear completely in any parent. Although most achieve partial resolutions to these painful emotions, it has been the authors' clinical experience that the mildest empathic probing of parents' feelings will inevitably reactivate intense repressed grief. This has been observed in parents of young children as well as in parents of deaf off-spring already in their middle years. Olshansky speaks of parents not only needing the opportunity to ventilate, clarify, and receive confirmation for the legitimacy of their feelings early on in the discovery of a child's disability but also potentially requiring such support at varying times throughout their lives.[7]

RESOLUTION OF FEELINGS TOWARD A CHILD'S DEAFNESS

As explained previously, the psychological implications of a child's deafness are only superficially understood by the parents. Such problems as educational methods can be resolved by conscious rational decisions. However, the deep psychological implications are not so easily resolved, especially those that prevail each time a new frustration taxes the parents' capacity to cope.

The disabled child is the ultimate challenge of the parents' capacity to cope with novel parental experiences. One effective way to cope is to look for advice and guidance to parents who have successfully raised children.

Todd contracted meningitis at 1 1/2 years of age. Despite the benefit of immediate educational intervention, use of hearing aids, and parental counseling, Todd functioned as a congenitally deaf child with a profound hearing loss. For example, his primary language was the language of signs. At the same time, Todd used his voice consistently in combination with the signs. Mr. and Mrs. S. made a satisfactory adjustment to the loss of their expectations of having a normal child and were asked to join a "buddy program" to share their experiences with other parents of newly diagnosed deaf children.

Lila contracted meningitis at the age of 2 and was diagnosed 6 months later as having a profound hearing loss. Mr. and Mrs. C. were obviously distressed at the diagnosis. They began to "shop" for an appropriate program. At the intake session, Lila appeared to be a happy, bright child who vocalized little. She communicated primarily through gestures, pointing, and facial expressions. Because of a number of similarities in family background, hospitalization of children and other experiences, Mrs. S. agreed to become a buddy and contact the C. family.

Significant gains can be made through parent-to-parent interaction with other hearing or deaf parents of deaf children. In the above case, Mrs. C was able to answer Mrs. S.'s questions on the basis of her experience with her deaf child. Mrs. S. was able to ask questions that she initially felt uncomfortable asking a professional. Mrs. S. commented that it was helpful to talk with another parent who shared similar experiences.

Educational programs sometimes do little to get parents together to share common feelings and experiences. Even worse, some have actively tried to prevent parents of young deaf children from interacting with parents of older deaf children. This shields the parents of the young child from hearing the obvious speech difficulties of the older deaf child and the regrets and bitterness of the other parents.[8]

Schlesinger and Meadow state that deaf children of hearing parents are characteristically deprived of contact with successful deaf adults. These lost experiences may negatively influence the ultimate self-concept of the child. "For if he only sees deaf children and never meets deaf adults, he may develop distorted expectations of what happens to deaf children grown up: Do they become like the hearing? Do they go into hiding? Do they disappear? Do they die?" The authors report on the research of Ervin-Tripp demonstrating the dramatic rise in self-esteem and self-achievement of disadvantaged children when successful adults of their own color or linguistic competence are introduced into their social and learning environments.[9]

When confronted with their child's deafness, parents begin a process that, if successful, allows them to abandon the hope of having a perfect and normal child. The original concept of the infant's future must be replaced with one based on realistic notions of the limits imposed by the disability. Only with a realistic appraisal of a deaf child's capacities is it possible for the parents to help that child achieve the maximum within his or her limitations.

It is only the rare parents who realize initially that their child's accomplishments will be significantly altered and limited by deafness in important ways. These parents waste no time in readjusting their notions of their child's capacities. More commonly, however, parents adopt positions based on unrealistic assessments of the child's capacities because of their own inability to relinquish fantasies of normality and perfection. Many things can lead them from their unwanted psychological burden. Perhaps the greatest comes from deaf children's visible similarities to hearing peers, except for deaf children with obvious physical handicaps. Among these similarities are vocal utterances similar to the sounds of young hearing children up to the age of 18 months, early play patterns that closely duplicate those of hearing children, and normal achievement of certain growth milestones such as creeping, walking, and running.

When considered in its own right, the promise of communication with the deaf child is a powerful and sustaining force. A sense of completeness and maternal success grows in the mother as she communicates with her child. As for the child, the absence of full communication with his or her parent leads to drastic alterations in development. It limits the child's capacity to develop feelings of closeness to the parent and subsequently to other members of the community. Gross cognitive deficiencies are inevitable. The child's limitations in communication with the parents prevents the parents from feeling that the child has successfully attained the growth milestones.

If the professional community offers the promise that meaningful communication through speech and lipreading will eventually occur between the parent and child, the parents are inclined to overlook their immediate inability to communicate effectively with their child. They will endure their child's meager achievements if their hope is for normal speech and communication. That is why some parents of 5-year-old deaf children can allow themselves to speak with pride of their child's spoken vocabulary even though it may be less than 5 words. The intense psychological need for a normal child leads the parents to deny this failure to develop communication. They do not see it as failure but as a promise of wonderful things to come. With the acquisition of the first word or the establishment of rudimentary gestural communication, there is temporary relief of parents' feelings. As the child matures, however, needs for complex communication skills rapidly increase. The differences between the deaf child and hearing peers become more noticeable. Parents' anxieties are reactivated.

This does not mean to imply that there is no communication if the parents subscribe to an oral-only approach. A limited communication usually does develop. It accounts in part for the parents' ability to tolerate this seemingly intolerable state. Through exchanges of feelings and inventive gestures, the parents and the child can communicate to some extent in areas of basic need. Love and anger are easily communicated without words, but the cognitive aspects integral to fully understanding and sharing those feelings and their causes are lost.

If adequate parent-child communication is not achieved early, parents may sink into a state of bitter resignation. The many potentialities the child had die unrealized. Parent and child are denied fulfillments that could have been theirs.

Perhaps the most difficult psychological burden to handle is the anger that the frustrations of deafness make an everyday part of life with a deaf child. It has been our observation that this anger is seldom if ever completely relieved.[10] Each new frustration in understanding and meeting the child's needs adds to the burden. This fact and its ramifications are central to understanding the role of total communication. A successful communicative vehicle for exchanging critical information as well as tender or angry feelings can provide profound gratification to parents. Improved communication reduces frustration, which in turn reduces anger.

As noted earlier, anger that is repressed rather than recognized eventually finds outlets. It can interfere with parents' objectivity in caring for their child, punctuating the relationship with angry outbursts. Schlesinger and Meadow noted that almost three times as many mothers of deaf children said they felt no discomfort about physical punishment of their children as compared to mothers of hearing children. The responses included mothers who admitted to spanking their children occasionally and felt that this was an acceptable method to control behavior. Some mothers, however, said flatly that spanking was the only disciplinary method that deaf children understood.[11] Parents who might discuss with their hearing child the ramifications of the child's behavior may instead physically punish the deaf child. The parents perceive that they are unable to control their deaf child's behavior by other than physical means. The parents' sense of helplessness and frustration may be alleviated when they feel in control of their deaf child.

Kind words that conceal angry feelings go unnoticed by deaf children. They must rely on nonverbal signs of communication such as facial displays of emotion. Deaf children depend upon expressions that parade across their parents' faces to reveal parental feelings and attitudes.

If the parents fail to resolve their feelings of grief, anger, guilt, and helplessness, they will be arrested in the earliest stage of psychological reaction to the child's deafness. This is the stage when psychological processes of denial and rationalization form the chief mode of handling the psychic pain caused by the child's deafness. Through such mechanisms parents may find temporary relief; they will now, however, find solutions to the more basic and enduring problems of developing communication. The deaf child is placed in the position of having to drag the parents along, demanding from them at each new stage a new adaptation which they are ill equipped to handle. Parents' early reactions to the discovery of deafness and their resolution of feelings about it influence all future decisions.

ROLE OF THE
PROFESSIONAL COMMUNITY

In reflecting on their experiences during the deaf child's infancy, many parents have voiced resentment toward members of the professional community who held back or misinformed them on the major issues about the deaf child's future adaptation. Parents may direct their angry feelings toward physicians who failed to fully heed the parents' forebodings of deafness, teachers who promised more than they could deliver, or audiologists who failed to give a clear message about the implications of the child's hearing loss.

The pediatrician or family practitioner is the professional usually consulted first when parents suspect that something is wrong with their infant. Many families report that pediatricians and family practitioners minimized their concerns, delaying definitive diagnosis to unspecified future times or misdiagnosing the hearing loss. Typically heard pediatrician clichés are "It's a phase," or "He'll outgrow it." Such suggestions and remarks are unfortunate and costly mistakes. They lead parents to procrastinate further over something that has already given them many months of uncertainty. Recollections of such experiences often form the core of angry indictments later hurled at the medical profession.

Unfortunately, most physicians — including ear, nose, and throat specialists — are unaware of the most basic issue in childhood deafness: how the condition interferes with the normal progression of the child's language and psychosocial development. Shah and Wong report that ". . . many studies like ours have found that parents are alert to their child's hearing impairment by about one year of age. Yet many physicians dismiss parental suspicions as invalid and regard neither parental observations nor a child's age as indications for referral and testing." Furthermore, Shah and Wong report that in their study "risk factors were present in 62% of cases. Common factors were rubella, birth problems (low birth weight, prematurity, placental insufficiency, strangulation, and convulsions), meningitis, a family history of deafness starting in childhood, Rh incompatibility, and hyperbilirubinemia. However, only 34.7% of the parents of such children had been advised of risk by their physicians at the appropriate time."[12]

Traditionally, even when physicians do refer children for testing, there is an assumption that once responsibility is handed over to the educational establishment, the future of the child is assured. To avoid being unwittingly drawn into this kind of delusion, physicians at large must be apprised of the real issues.

Professionals must recognize that parents are often ready to accept anything that promises to resolve their unhappy feelings during the early stages of discovery. Whether hearing aid dealer or physician, the first professional to whom the parents speak about their child is being asked for much more than a diagnosis. The parents' grief and anxiety are at their height. Their uncritical attitude is related to factors not within their conscious awareness. Despite their repeated acts of denial and rationalization, the parents have been unable to rid themselves of the belief that the child is deaf. There are few professionals who are prepared or who will attempt to meet the parents' primary need: to discuss, ventilate, and understand their feelings toward their deaf child. It is not uncommon for the busy physician or audiologist to feel that his or her responsibility has been fulfilled once the diagnosis of irreversible deafness has been established. Yet this is the parents' time of greatest need.

Professionals should consciously reckon with their own feelings over having to tell parents something that will hurt and upset them. Usually they do not and thus are often inclined to assuage the parents' anguish by offering sympathy. Such offerings lead at best to temporary relief and inevitably delay more effective procedures.

Issues discussed by Simon Olshansky regarding parents of mentally retarded children can be applied to other handicapping conditions such as deafness. He states that the helping professions have somewhat belabored the tendency of the parent to deny the reality of the child's mental deficiency. Few workers have reported what is probably a more frequent occurrence, the parent's tendency to deny their chronic sorrow. This tendency is often reinforced by the professional's habit of viewing chronic sorrow as a neurotic manifestation rather than as a natural and understandable response to a tragic fact . . . a parent's experiencing chronic sorrow does not preclude his deriving satisfaction and joy from his child's modest achievements in growth and development.[13]

CONCLUSION

When parents have been informed that their child is deaf, the feelings of grief must be acknowledged following diagnosis. Mobilization of constructive mental health resources is sufficient and the best form of acknowledgment. Referral to centers providing comprehensive services is essential. It is the responsibility of the mental health professional to provide these direct services to the parents, as well as to enlighten other concerned professionals about the relevant psychological phenomena of this period so that they in turn will be more able to manage these issues with sensitivity and sophistication.

We must recognize that, even when parents initially receive services from sensitive and competent professionals, there may be difficulties later in the child's life. Even professionals directly related to the field of deafness may be inadequately trained or lack the appropriate materials and equipment for the population they serve. For example, in one city, a state agency providing services to deaf children and young adults did not have a TTY with which to communicate with many of their clients, including the deaf parents of deaf children. In the same city, a major university was graduating audiologists unskilled in the language of signs. When a hearing man was asked to interpret the results of his deaf wife's audiological evaluation, he refused to do so. He bluntly told the audiologist that to work effectively with her clients she must learn sign language.

As we have demonstrated, the manner in which the parents interact with the child and act on his or her behalf is determined by many different factors. As a consequence, team intervention is appropriate. Such a team ideally should be comprised of professionals in education, audiology, psychology, social work, psychiatry, neurology, and other medical or related services such as ophthalmology or physical medicine.

Universally, those who have constructed programs for young disabled children have observed that, unless the parents' emotional needs are adequately served, the programs have limited benefit for the children. Parents must receive services that afford them the knowledge, understanding, and attitudes to exercise proficiently their responsibilities as the primary decision makers, care givers, teachers, and advocates for their own children. Only through these comprehensive services will handicapped infants or children and their families overcome or compensate for the constraints arising from deafness.[14]

In this chapter, we have discussed the unfolding of childhood deafness and its effect upon the family. The goal is to help parents achieve a flexible relationship with their deaf child, which is impossible without adequate communication. If this goal is achieved, parents can provide the needed link between the child and the world beyond home.

A close correlation exists between parents' early reactions to the discovery of deafness in their child and their future handling of the child. Successful adaptations to childhood deafness are still rare today because of the scarcity of total rehabilitation programs. As a consequence, deaf children become progressively more isolated from their families and from the hearing community as well. The reactions that mire the family in bitterness and resentment can be prevented by early enlightened professional intervention.

REFERENCES

1. Mendelsohn, J. Z. (1981). The parent-professional: A personal view. In *Deafness and mental health*. Stein, L. K., Mindel, E. D., and Jabaley, T. (Eds.), (p. 40). New York: Grune & Stratton.
2. Schlesinger, H. S. and Meadow, K. P. (1972). Sound and sign: Childhood deafness and mental health. Berkeley: University of California Press.
3. Cholden, L. S. (1958). *A psychiatrist works with blindness.* New York: American Foundation for the Blind. Hamburg, D. A. (1953, March). *Psychological adaptive processes in life threatening injuries.* Paper presented at the Symposium on Stress, Walter Reed Medical Center, Washington, D.C.

4. Oxford, D. R., and Aponte, J. F. (1967). Distortion of disability and effect on family life. *Journal of the American Academy of Child Psychiatry, 6,* 499–511. Butani, P. (1974). Reactions of mothers to the birth of an anomalous infant: A review of the literature. *Maternal Child Nursing Journal, 3,* 64–65.

5. Vernon, M. (1969). Sociological and Psychological factors associated with profound hearing loss. *Journal of Speech and Hearing Research, 12,* 541–563.

6. Mindel, E. D. (1968). A child psychiatrist looks at deafness. *Deaf American, 20,* 15–19.

7. Olshansky, S. (1962). Chronic sorrow: A response to having a mentally defective child. *Child Social Casework, 43* (4), 191–195.

8. Mindel, E.D. *Op. cit.*

9. Schlesinger, H. S., and Meadow, K. P. *Op. cit.,* 17–18.

10. Grinker, R. G. (Ed.) (1969). *Psychiatric diagnosis, therapy, and research on the psychotic deaf.* Final Report Grant No. RD-2407-S, Social Rehabilitation Service, Department of Health, Education, and Welfare (Available from Dr. Grinker, Michael Reese Hospital, 2959 S. Ellis, Chicago, IL 60616).

11. Schlesinger, H. S., and Meadow, K. P. *Op. cit.,* 103–104.

12. Shah, C. P., and Wong, D. (1979). Failure in early detection of hearing impairment in preschool children. *Journal of the Division of Early Childhood, 1,* (1), 36.

13. Olshansky, S. *Op. cit.,* 191.

14. Garland, C., Stone, N. W., Swanson, J., and Woodruff, G. (Eds.) (1981). Early intervention for children with special needs and their families: Findings and recommendations. WESTAR Series Paper No. 11, Contract No. 300-77-0508, Washington, D.C.: Office of Special Education.

CHAPTER 2

The Primary Causes of Deafness

McCay Vernon

The major causes of deafness also may cause brain damage, heart defects, visual problems, or other congenital anomalies. Thus, the disease process causing deafness may have other far-reaching effects on behavior and physical well-being.

Suspicion that a child was born deaf may arise if there is a family history of deafness or if during her pregnancy the mother contracted maternal rubella. Severe neonatal jaundice due to incompatibility between the blood of the mother (Rh negative) and her infant (Rh positive) may damage the hearing apparatus before or just after birth. In such cases physicians should inform parents of the possibility of deafness and arrange for audiological evaluation. Hearing loss may also be due to a serious infection occurring after birth that affects the brain or its covering membranes. If the onset is prior to the time the child has started speaking in sentences — about 18 months to 2 years — the loss may not be immediately recognized. If it occurs after this age, when the child has begun to communicate verbally, the deafness will be apparent immediately. Milder hearing losses are not so readily identified.

DISEASE PROCESSES PRIOR TO BIRTH

The major current cause of congenital deafness is genetic.[1] Rubella is still a prominent cause, despite the development of effective vaccines.[2] Deafness in offspring is anticipated most often when one or both parents are deaf due to hereditary causes. However, today most deaf adults do not know the reason for their own deafness. In fact, establishing the cause of deafness, even with the current emphasis on birth defects, is often extremely difficult.

Heredity

Genetic factors have been the leading cause of deafness throughout this century except during certain epidemic periods of rubella. Generally, 40 to 60 percent of all deafness is attributed to heredity.[3]

It often astonishes professionals in the rehabilitation of deaf persons to discover that 90 percent of genetic deafness is carried by a recessive gene. This is especially surprising in cases where there may be no known deafness in the immediate family. The lottery of genetics is such that, although this recessive gene for deafness is present in approximately 1 out of 10 persons, only 6 children per 10,000 are deafened genetically.[3] The recessive gene in one parent has to be matched by one in the other parent, if a recessive trait is to appear in their child.

Children deafened through hereditary causes are less likely to have other defects than are children deafened from nongenetic causes. As a group, the genetically deaf do better in school.[4] There is also evidence to suggest that, as a group, they may have slightly higher intelligence test scores than deaf and hearing children generally have.[5,6] Paradoxically, however, parents generally loath to accept the fact that their child's deafness is of genetic origin. They react to such a diagnosis as if it stigmatizes them. In view of the commonness of recessive gene carriers and the excellent achievement record of genetically deaf children, this attitude, though understandable, is certainly unnecessary.

Where genetic deafness is suspected or established, the family should take two important steps. First, competent genetic counseling should be sought in order that all family members can be made fully aware of the probabilities for deafness in future offspring. Second, regular and complete ophthalmological examinations should be sought because, of the 60 plus known forms of genetic deafness, there are 10 that involve both hearing loss and visual problems.[3]

Rubella

Between 1963 and 1965, a rubella epidemic raged across the United States.[7] It resulted in the birth of more handicapped children than did the thalidomide disaster. Rehabilitation programs for deaf youth are still serving a huge number of offspring of this epidemic. Whereas rubella usually causes about 10 percent of deafness in children, schools that served youngsters born during the 1963 to 1965 period reported a 40 to 80 percent prevalence of postrubella cases of deafness (i.e., over one half of all deaf children born during the 1963–65 period were deafened by rubella).

Rubella is an incipient disease. A mother will be aware of the illness if she has developed a rash, swollen lymph nodes in her neck, and low-grade fever. However, in about 40 percent of the cases the disease does not come to actual clinical definition. Thus, many mothers are unaware of the rubella infection they had during gestation.[8] When the rash occurs, it is typically evanescent. By the time the mother appears for examination by her physician two or three days later, it may have already disappeared.

Although the rubella virus usually causes only a mild illness in the mother, it can seriously affect a developing fetus. Deafness is the most frequent handicap, but visual problems (cataracts and/or retinal damage), lowered intelligence, or heart defects can also occur. Studies indicate that 85 to 90 percent of postrubella infants suffer significant physical damage during gestation.[1,9]

The period of greatest danger to the fetus is the first 3 months of pregnancy, but damage can occur even if the mother is infected within a few weeks prior to conception, or as late as the eighth or ninth month.[1,9] Rarely is there significant damage to infants infected after birth.

The rubella virus is not necessarily eliminated from the infant's tissue after birth. It has been cultured in adults 25 years after prenatal infection. It can remain within various cells of the body and continue to cause cellular damage for an as yet undetermined period of time. For example, some rubella children have come down with juvenile diabetes in their teens due to the latent manifestation of the virus.

Vaccines that give promise of eventually eliminating rubella as a major cause of deafness are now available.[10] Potential undesirable side effects as well as the effectiveness of these vaccines to control epidemics remain as concerns.

Regular physical and audiological examinations are important for postrubella youngsters. Since the probability of other problems such as poor vision, heart trouble, diabetes, and neurological damage are high, these possibilities must be thoroughly investigated by pediatricians, ophthalmologists, and other appropriate specialists.[7,11] Sometimes the parent must assume responsibility for seeking specialized examinations for the child because the family doctor may not always detect subtle visual or neurological difficulties.

DISEASES OF THE PERINATAL PERIOD

There are several prominent causes of deafness related to this period. These are prematurity, sexually transmitted diseases, and blood-type (Rh-factor) incompatibility.[12]

Parents cannot be expected to anticipate deafness in a premature infant or one having blood-type incompatibility. A pediatrician may advise parents of such a possibility, especially in the case of a jaundiced infant; however, most physicians and other professionals do not wish to alarm parents unduly. In any case, physicians should consider these infants as high risk and should follow them accordingly.[12]

Sexually Transmitted Diseases

Changes in sex practices in the United States have led to an epidemic of sexually transmitted diseases. Such diseases as herpes simplex and cytomegalovirus (CMV) may cause deafness and other defects in children born to infected mothers. Insufficient data exist to predict actual numbers of cases but an estimated 5 to 10 percent of CMV-infected children have hearing losses.[11] Many children deafened due to sexually transmitted diseases have severe multiple handicaps.

Premature Birth

It has been established that four times as many deaf as hearing children are born prematurely. (The World Health Organization has defined a premature infant as one weighing no more than 5 pounds 8 ounces at birth.) Approximately 17 percent school-aged deaf youth were born prematurely.[5,6,14]

While the prematurity itself is rarely a direct cause of hearing loss, its association with deafness deserves consideration. This is particularly true when the child is born prematurely and no other cause of deafness can be isolated. Conditions such as lack of oxygen and cerebral hemorrhage, which can damage the nervous system, are more common among premature than among full-term infants and can cause deafness.

Children known to have been born prematurely should be regarded as high risks for hearing loss. If deafness is diagnosed, thorough physical examinations should be made to check for other problems, especially those involving vision, the central nervous system, and the heart, which have a heightened probability in children known to be both deaf and premature.

Rh-Factor Incompatibility

Certain genetic combinations of blood types in parents result in blood incompatibilities between mother and child during pregnancy. One of these occurs when Rh-negative mothers have Rh-positive fetuses. The mother's antibodies may cross the placenta and enter the bloodstream of the fetus, destroying the blood cells and leading to severe jaundice in the newborn baby. When this occurs, death may result at or soon after birth. An exchange transfusion can prevent death, but if not performed soon enough, products of blood cell destruction are deposited in the brain.[13] Of those who survive, a large proportion is deaf, and many may additionally have cerebral palsy or problems in language development.[5,6]

Advances in medical science may soon eliminate Rh incompatibility as a significant cause of deafness.[15] Postnatal and in utero blood transfusions can prevent some of the effects of this incompatibility. In addition, a special gamma globulin has been developed that when administered to an Rh-negative mother after the birth of her first Rh-positive child will eliminate the destructive anti-Rh-positive antibodies formed during pregnancy, thus giving a second Rh-positive child no greater chance of being affected than the first child.

CHILDHOOD DISEASES

The destructive processes of diseases such as meningitis and encephalitis can cause deafness. There may also be damage to parts of the brain crucial to language learning.[5,6,15] The child thus affected has special problems in subsequent language development.

The period of maximum language growth is between the ages of 2 and 4. Children deafened after this critical period generally retain at least basic mastery of syntax.

A child who freely communicated with his or her parents until the onset of meningitis or encephalitis, and who was then deprived of this communication, has difficult adjustment problems. Fear, due to having almost died of the illness may accompany the loss of hearing. Similarly, the near loss of their child can leave parents feeling they must now treat the child with special care.

Meningitis

Approximately 10 percent of deafness originating in childhood is caused by meningitis, an inflammation of the meninges, the protective coverings of the brain and spinal cord. The disease deafens an estimated 3 to 5 percent of the children who contract it. Many organisms can infect the meninges; the chance that deafness will develop depends in part upon which organism has caused the meningitis.[5,16]

A major clinical problem of meningitis is that symptoms such as headache, stiff neck, or fever cannot be readily diagnosed in infants and young children. Infants cannot specify the location of their discomfort to the doctor or their parents and can only react to the situation by irritability or tears; hence, the disease is often not diagnosed immediately. Sometimes it is only when stronger symptoms manifest — a fever above 100 degrees, a seizure, or a coma — that the child is taken to a doctor or hospitalized, and the laboratory tests required for definitive diagnosis are made. The delay in instituting therapy may lead to deafness. The fact that premature and very young infants are especially susceptible to meningitis compounds this problem.

The development of antibiotics and their introduction into clinical medicine has greatly improved the survival rate for most victims of the disease, and at the same time has changed the characteristics of postmeningitic children[5,16] Previously, very young children, especially premature infants and those less than one month of age, died from the disease. Now they survive in significant numbers and frequently have residual effects of sufficient magnitude to interfere with normal adaptation. (Examples of clinically detectable effects on the nervous system are learning disorders, muscle weakness, paralysis, and deafness.[12])

Because of this and because the disease frequently causes additional neurological damage, our educational methods for these children must change correspondingly.

Encephalitis

The viral organisms that cause such diseases as mumps and the 2-week measles may subsequently invade the brain, causing encephalitis.[12] One result may be deafness. When this occurs, there are often other disabilities such as learning difficulties and behavior disorders.

MISCONCEPTIONS ABOUT CAUSES OF DEAFNESS

Not uncommonly members of the lay public consider "brain fever," a blow on the head, or a high fever that "burned up the nerve" to be the reason for a child's deafness. It appears logical to connect these events to the deafness, since nearly all parents can recall times when their child received a hard blow on the head or had a high fever. This reasoning seems valid when the deafness is discovered at 2 or 3 years of age and when there is no other known cause.

Fever alone does not cause hearing loss, nor is a blow to the head likely to do so unless it is severe enough to fracture the bones of the skull that protect the auditory mechanisms. These mechanisms are well protected by the skull, and furthermore are located on both sides of the head. Fractures damaging hearing in both ears simultaneously would be a rare occurrence. Unless such damage or a specific disease such as meningitis is identified, brain fever, burned-up nerves, or falling from the cradle are unlikely explanations. At best, these are inexact reasons for a child's deafness.

It is helpful for parents to know the cause of their child's hearing loss. Although the sensorineural loss itself generally is unalterable, the knowledge will generally reduce the parents' tendency to blame themselves. Furthermore, establishing the etiology may prevent the birth of additional deaf children and be of value in treating and understanding the child. It is especially important for the deaf child to have frequent, thorough medical checkups by a pediatrician and otologist. Neurologists and ophthalmologists should also be consulted to provide care for any coexisting nervous system or visual defects.

REFERENCES

1. Vernon, M., Grieve, B. J., and Shaver, K. A. (1980). Handicapping conditions in the congenital rubella syndrome. *American Annals of the Deaf, 125*, 993–997.
2. Trybus, R. J., Karchmer, M. A. Kerstetter, P. P. and Hicks, W. (1980). The demographics of deafness resulting from maternal rubella. *American Annals of the Deaf, 125*, 997–984.
3. Shaver, K., and Vernon, M. (1978). Genetics and hearing loss: An overview for professions. *Rehabilitation Literature, 4*, (2), 6–10.
4. Moores, D. F. (1978). *Educating the deaf: Psychology, principles and practices.* Boston: Houghton Mifflin.
5. Vernon, M. (1982). Multiply handicapped deaf children. In D. Tweedie and E. H. Shroyer (Eds.), *The multiply handicapped hearing impaired: Identification and instruction.* Washington, D.C.: Gallaudet Press.
6. Vernon, M. (1969). *Multiply handicapped deaf children: Medical, educational and psychological considerations.* (Research Monograph). Reston, VA: Council of Exceptional Children.
7. Hardy, B., Monif, G. R. G., and Sever, J. L. (1966). Studies in congenital rubella, Baltimore 1964–1965. II: Clinic and virologic. *Bulletin of the Johns Hopkins Hospital, 118*, 97–108.
8. Karmody, C. S. (1969). Asymptomatic maternal rubella and congenital deafness. *Archives of Otolaryngology, 89*, 62–68.
9. Chess, S., and Fernandez, P. (1980). Neurologic damage and behavior disorder in rubella children. *American Annals of the Deaf, 125*, 998–1001.
10. Preblud, J. P., Hinman, A. R., and Herrman, K. L. (1980). An evaluation of the United States rubella immunization program. *American Annals of the Deaf, 125*, 968–976.
11. Vernon, M., and Hicks, D. (1980). Overview of rubella, herpes simplex, cytomegalovirus, and other viral diseases: Their relationships to deafness. *American Annals of the Deaf, 125*, 529–534.
12. Mindel, E. D., and Vernon, M. (1971). *They grow in silence,* Silver Spring, MD: National Association for Deaf Press.
13. Paine, R. S. Kernicterus. *Clinical Proceedings, 24*, 1968, 37–47.
14. Vernon, M. (1967b). Prematurity and deafness: The magnitude and nature of the problem among deaf children. *Exceptional Child, 38*, 289–298.
15. Vernon, M. (1981). The decade of the eighties: Significant trends and developments for the hearing impaired. *Rehabilitation Literature, 42* 2–7.
16. Vernon, M. (1967a). Meningitis and deafness. *Larynoscope, 77*, 1856–1874.

CHAPTER 3

Audiology and the Hearing-Impaired Child: Current Status and Future Needs

Noel D. Matkin

A growing body of research has highlighted the pervasive effects of hearing losses upon language development.[1] Even losses of a mild degree that previously were not considered handicapping can cause considerable language delay. As a result, there is increased concern relative to early identification and referral of all children at risk for hearing impairment.

A number of developments during the past decade has made it possible to significantly improve the quality of audiologic services available to hearing-impaired children and their families. Specifically, there is now a variety of clinical techniques and materials to use when assessing the hearing of young children and infants. This battery of tests will be discussed in some detail later in this chapter. A further noteworthy development is improved hearing aid technology that now makes it possible to fit more children with small ear-level instruments having good electroacoustic flexibility, high gain, and acceptable fidelity.

Although the developments described above are encouraging, a number of persisting problems merit discussion. First, screening programs to assure early identification are lacking in most communities, especially during the period between discharge from the newborn hospital nursery and kindergarten. Second, many physicians are poorly educated relative to early developmental milestones in hearing, language, and speech. Consequently, parents frequently are assured that there is no cause for concern, only to find months or even years later that an educationally significant hearing loss was the basis of delay in development of communication skills. Finally, audiologic findings often are not integrated into educational planning. As a result of these persisting problems, many hearing-impaired children are still identified relatively late. On one hand, the educational program often is not individualized to assure maximum utilization of residual hearing, even after a comprehensive audiologic evaluation. On the other hand, the limitations imposed by the hearing loss are not considered in program planning; as a consequence, unrealistic levels of expectation relative to potential auditory function are set.

Three basic axioms underlie the following discussion: (1) hearing is the primary modality by which speech and language is normally and most efficiently acquired; (2) the preschool years represent the optimal period for language learning; and (3) the majority of hearing-impaired children possess sufficient residual hearing to merit hearing aid utilization from an early age, regardless of the educational approach, be it aural/oral or total communication.

EARLY IDENTIFICATION

As the pervasive effects of even mild and moderate hearing losses upon cognitive, language, and communication development have been recognized, the importance of early identification and intervention increasingly has been stressed.[2,3] Recognition of the preschool years as the prime language learning period, during which the foundations are laid for verbal communication and subsequent academic achievement, has resulted in early identification programs being viewed as an essential public health priority.[4] Further, studies reporting anatomical changes resulting from sensory deprivation in both the central visual and auditory pathways of young animals are cited as further evidence to justify early intervention, including the use of amplification, with hearing-impaired infants.[5,6] Finally, there is evidence that full-time hearing aid use is enhanced by introducing amplification as early as possible.[7]

Although the rationale for early intervention typically has focused on the potential benefits for the hearing-impaired infant or child, the benefits for parents should also be considered. The anxiety, frustration, and depression often encountered in parents prior to a definitive diagnosis may undermine optimal parenting. Thus, undue delays in identification and intervention may result in developmental deficits not only directly from the hearing loss, but also indirectly through unenlightened parenting. Such deficits may never be fully remedied. In short, intervention programs should be designed to support the family, as well as the child.

In 1964 and 1965, the rubella epidemic caused a heightened sense of urgency among physicians, clinicians, and educators to detect infants with developmentally significant hearing losses. The recommended approach, at that time, was to assess the auditory responsiveness of all newborn with a neurometer, a hand-held signal generator.[8] The test signal typically used was a high-intensity, high-frequency warble tone (90 dB SPL at 3000 Hz). Those infants who did not demonstrate an observable response upon testing were labeled "at risk for hearing loss" and subsequently were scheduled for later detailed audiologic testing. Follow-up study of these mass screening programs revealed a number of shortcomings. Approximately 1 in 1,500 to 2,000 infants was identified as having a severe or profound bilateral hearing impairment, but many infants who initially failed the hearing screening were later found to have normal hearing sensitivity.[9] A substantial number of newborns with mild and moderate sensorineural hearing deficits may have passed screening because they responded to the high-intensity test signal used.[10] After considering both the high number of false positives and false negatives, as well as the relatively low yield from such screening, a study committee comprised of representatives from the American Speech and Hearing Association, the American Academy of Pediatrics, and the American Academy of Ophthalmology and Otolaryngology was convened. This committee could not recommend initiation of mass neonatal screening programs except in research designed to further refine and improve the approach.[11]

As a result of this 1970 resolution, attention shifted to the development of high-risk registers, with hearing screening limited to those infants deemed to be at risk in view of their familial or medical histories. The factors most frequently cited as putting an infant at risk for hearing loss include familial history of deafness; physical abnormalities of the ear, nose, and throat; maternal infection such as rubella; high bilirubin count, as with Rh incompatibility; and low birth weight, often with hypoxia. The reported prevalence of hearing loss among high-risk neonates is 1 in 40.[12] Use of a high-risk questionnaire limits screening to approximately 7 percent of all newborns in this country, thereby reducing time, effort, and cost.

In the last few years, the focus of most direct screening programs has been infants placed in neonatal intensive care units (NICUs). Clinical investigations using either brainstem audiometry or the Crib-o-Gram automatic screening procedure have revealed that approximately 2 to 10 percent of such babies are found to have significant sensorineural impairments.[13,14]

Neonatal hearing screening programs concentrating on the NICU population are laudable, yet their shortcomings must be recognized. A significant number of newborns should be considered at risk for hearing loss, but are essentially healthy babies and thus are not in intensive care units. Included in this group are most infants with a family history of hearing loss due to dominant genetic transmission. Most endogenous or familial hearing losses among newborns are due to recessive rather than dominant genetic transmission; thus, both parents have normal hearing and there may not be a family history of hearing loss. Again, such babies will not be cared for in an NICU. Many cases of maternal prenatal infections, including those due to rubella and cytomegalovirus (and certain other sexually transmitted diseases), may be subclinical so that there is no prenatal history of illness to suggest that such babies are at risk. Finally, it is estimated that approximately 30 percent of all pediatric sensorineural hearing losses are acquired postnatally, and are not congenital.[15] Thus, hearing screening must be considered as an essential ongoing component of preschool health care. Otherwise children may not be identified until pure tone screening is conducted upon entry into kindergarten, or even later.

Parents typically express their initial concern about developmental delays to the child's physician, who may ignore them. It is imperative that pediatricians and family practitioners become better informed about early signs of hearing loss, especially speech-language delay.* Physicians also must be encouraged to respond positively to parents' observations that something is different about their child's development and refer the child for an evaluation of sensory function and development. The frequent recommendation to "wait and see if he outgrows it" is an inappropriate response. Even in cases of profound bilateral hearing loss, a delay in diagnosis of a year to 18 months after parents initially express their concern to the family physician is not unusual.[16,17] One recent survey of parents revealed that 56 percent initially had been assured, most often by pediatricians, that their child probably did not have a hearing impairment.[18]

CLINICAL PHILOSOPHY

There are four essential features of a comprehensive pediatric audiologic evaluation for a child at risk for a hearing loss. Each feature must be given equal consideration for the audiologic evaluation to be comprehensive.

1. Completion of a case history, including developmental as well as medical information
2. Observations of the child's auditory and language behavior in both unstructured and structured activities
3. Clinical testing, including not only detailed measures of hearing, but appropriate screening in the major developmental areas (cognition, motor, language, and social)
4. Parent-child programming, including education, guidance, and counseling.

The time and effort expended in each area will depend on the nature and severity of the child's disorder. For example, the procedures may be abbreviated when it becomes apparent that the primary problem is related to middle ear effusion, requiring active medical management and only audiologic monitoring. In contrast, when a sensorineural hearing impairment is identified in which long-term remedial and educational planning, including hearing aid use, is required, all four features of the audiologic evaluation should be extensive.

Information obtained from the case history, behavioral observations, and direct clinical testing should yield a cohesive clinical diagnosis of the child's level of auditory function, as well

---

*Young children who have normal hearing but who are mentally retarded, autistic, or brain damaged initially may appear to be hearing impaired, since they do not respond consistently and appropriately to sounds in their environment.

as current strengths and limitations. Otherwise, detailed feedback to the parents and the formulation of a rehabilitative plan should be postponed until further evaluation has been undertaken and the apparent discrepancies have been resolved.

The audiologist, who often is the first nonmedical professional to interact with the child and the family, is in a unique position to facilitate (or, conversely, to impede) comprehensive remedial and educational planning. If screening measures used during the evaluation suggest that developmental delays in addition to those imposed by a hearing loss exist, it is the audiologist's responsibility to work with both the parents and the referral source to ensure that a comprehensive multidisciplinary assessment is undertaken in order to provide that child with the most appropriate program at the earliest possible age. Unfortunately, some clinicians see their only responsibility as obtaining information about the child's hearing status. Such a constricted viewpoint can significantly delay needed additional referrals and early intervention. With current demographic data indicating that approximately one third of all children with sensorineural hearing losses may have one or more additional handicapping conditions, it becomes critical that each audiological evaluation in a pediatric setting be viewed as diagnostic in nature.[19] In my clinical experience, an increasing number of children with marked developmental delays, but ultimately found to have normal hearing, are referred for hearing tests. Again, the parents need specific guidance and direction regarding the need for further developmental evaluation.

Once a hearing loss has been identified, periodic reevaluations should be scheduled so that the initial audiologic impression can be refined as more detailed information is obtained. Another reason for scheduling reevaluations is that many sensorineural hearing losses are progressive, necessitating hearing aid and educational program modification. Additionally, any child, especially during the preschool years, may develop middle ear infections, which, if undetected, can impose additional hearing loss and limit the benefits of both the hearing aid and educational programs. Finally, by evaluating changes in auditory and communicative function over time, the family and professionals can assure that the impact of the hearing loss is being minimized as much as possible by appropriate rehabilitation. Six-month reevaluations during the preschool years and yearly appointments during the elementary school years are recommended.

AUDIOLOGICAL EVALUATION

The primary objectives of an audiological evaluation, regardless of the client's age, are threefold. First, basic to all subsequent measures is a description of the hearing loss in each ear relative to degree, type, and configuration. Traditionally, the degree of the hearing impairment is first assessed with pure tones and then confirmed using a speech signal. Pure tones are presented via earphones at octave intervals across a range which covers the acoustic spectrum of speech (250–8000 Hz), including vowels, voiced consonants (e.g., b, z, d, g) and voiceless consonants (e.g., p, s, t, k). By recording on an audiogram the lowest intensity at which an individual responds to each test signal and then comparing these response levels (or thresholds) with those of average young listeners, both the degree and the configuration of the hearing loss can be determined.* Although universal guidelines for classifying hearing losses have not been adopted, there is general agreement as to a classification system. Rather than describe a hearing loss as a percentage of loss, most clinicians use descriptive terms relative to the degree of hearing loss based on the pure tone audiogram (Table 3–1). While it is dangerous to generalize, Table 3–1 highlights the problems often encountered at different degrees of the hearing loss.

The audiogram in Figure 3–1 would be described as illustrative of a bilateral, moderate impairment with a sloping configuration. This individual would not hear soft conversational speech (approximately 35 dB). Further, average conversational speech (50 dB), while being detected, could not be understood through hearing alone. In contrast, the audiogram in Figure 3–2 reflects a bilateral, profound impairment with a fragmentary configuration. A child with this impairment would not hear average conversational speech. Although loud speech would be detected, it could not be understood, because the consonants (which fall into the high-frequency range) would not be audible.

---

*Many physicians, as part of a routine physical examination, assess the patient's hearing with tuning forks. Tuning forks, like audiometers, are calibrated to emit pure tones at various octave frequencies (256, 512, 1024 Hz, etc.). The accuracy of such hearing tests is directly related to the patient's ability to follow verbal directions and make rather complex loudness judgments. Unfortunately, young children do not have either the cognitive or linguistic skills to reliably respond to this medical approach to hearing testing; results from tuning fork tests can be quite misleading and can result in further delays in identification or in misclassification of the child's problem.

Table 3–1. *Problems Associated with Degree of Hearing Loss*

Degree of Hearing Loss	Pure Tone Average	Associated Problems
Borderline Normal	11 to 25 dB	Will rarely be detected without formal audiometric testing. Child often accused of not paying attention or daydreaming.
Mild	26 to 45 dB	Will have difficulty hearing soft speech or hearing at a distance. Performance in school will vary without a hearing aid, depending on distance from teacher and classroom noise and lighting. A language delay of 1 to 2 years is not uncommon.
Moderate	46 to 65 dB	Will understand conversations without amplification only at close distance and if structure of language and vocabulary are controlled. Early attention to oral language development will be needed as delays of 3 or more years are often encountered.
Severe	66 to 85 dB	Will not perceive normal conversation without hearing aid or auditory training unit. Will need either resource services or special classes, depending on language skills including vocabulary development and usage, as well as reading and writing abilities.
Profound	86 dB or More	Will occasionally hear loud environmental sounds without amplification, but often responds instead to vibrations. Will need early and intensive program for deaf children with emphasis on concept development, all language and academic skills, both receptively and expressively.

Note: Adapted from *Relationship of Hearing Impairment to Educational Needs* by R. J. Bernero and H. Bothwell (1966). Illinois Department of Public Health and Office of the Superintendent of Public Instruction.

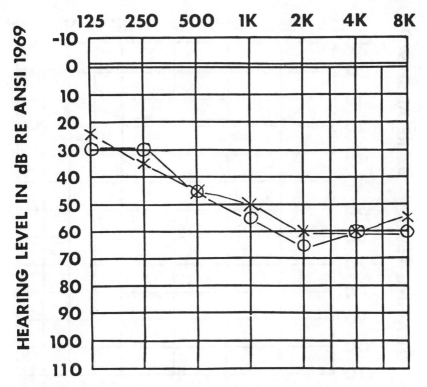

Figure 3–1.   *The audiogram of a child with a moderate sloping sensorineural hearing impairment in both ears, of unknown etiology (0 = right ear response; x = left ear response).*

If the pure tone findings are reliable, the threshold for speech should be in the same general category of hearing loss.

Once the degree and configuration of a hearing loss is determined, the next objective is to ascertain whether the impairment is due to dysfunction in the conductive mechanism (outer and/or middle ear) or in the deep sensorineural structures of the ear (inner ear and/or auditory nerve). This determination is essential to management, because the majority of conductive impairments can be eliminated through either medical or surgical treatment. In contrast, sensorineural impairments are not correctable. Their impact must be minimized through rehabilitation, including hearing aid use and, in the case of children, special education.

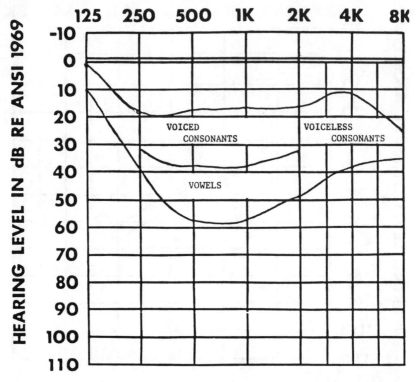

Figure 3–2. *The audiogram of a child with a profound fragmentary sensorineural hearing impairment in both ears following hospitalization with meningitis at 17 months of age (0 = right ear response; x = left ear response).*

In recent years, growing concern has been expressed about two subgroups of children. Some children who developed middle ear problems in infancy continue to experience repeated bouts of otitis media, with an accompanying hearing loss.[20] There is growing evidence that, although such hearing losses fluctuate and rarely exceed a mild degree of impairment, significant delays in language and learning may result.[21] This observation has stimulated considerable research relative to improved medical treatment and educational management. However, most conductive hearing losses are eliminated with otologic management. The second subgroup who merit mention are children with an undetected conductive hearing loss superimposed upon a sensorineural hearing impairment (i.e., those with a mixed type of hearing loss). A recent othologic study conducted in a school for the deaf revealed a surprisingly high prevalence of middle ear pathology.[22] Of approximately 400 students, 29 percent were found to have middle ear problems at some time during the school year. Such impairments, undetected, may impose additional health and educational problems.

Two audiological procedures are utilized to ascertain the type of hearing loss. First, pure tones are delivered via a bone conduction vibrator through the mastoid bone to the inner ear. If the loss is sensorineural, the same degree and configuration of hearing loss will be observed as that via earphone presentations. In contrast, normal bone conduction findings indicate an intact inner ear and auditory nerve. In such a case, the dysfunction is due to a problem in the outer or, usually, the middle ear.

The second clinical approach used to assess the type of hearing loss is impedance audiometry. This newer procedure, which does not require the active cooperation of the client, is widely used with children. Although space prohibits detailed discussion of the technical aspects of this procedure, a brief description follows.

The impedance procedure does not measure hearing, but rather the efficiency with which an auditory signal is conducted through the middle ear system. If the middle ear mechanism is functioning properly, the majority of sound is transmitted across the bony bridge of three tiny bones in the middle ear once the eardrum is set into vibration. However, even in a healthy ear, a minute amount of sound is reflected back toward the outer ear after striking the eardrum. With appropriate instrumentation, this reflected energy can be measured. A number of middle ear conditions, including either negative pressure or fluid associated with a middle ear infection, will impede movement of the eardrum. Consequently, the reflected energy, which is measured and plotted on a chart (the tympanogram), will be substantially different than that of a normal subject. With this method, young children having middle ear conditions can be detected with a minimum of time, effort, and cost, and early referral to a physician is feasible.

The same instrumentation can be used to determine whether the presentation of a very loud pure tone causes the tiny muscles in the middle ear to contract. In the normal ear, there is a middle ear muscle reflex in response to a loud sound, much as the pupil of the eye contracts to a bright light. Assessing whether the acoustic reflex is present, elevated, or absent provides further diagnostic information regarding type and degree of hearing loss. An excellent discussion of impedance measures, including instrumentation, clinical procedures, and interpretation of findings can be found in *Basic Audiologic Evaluation.*[23]

A common misconception leading to late identification and management is that the hearing status of preschool children and infants cannot be reliably measured. Systematic clinical investigations have revealed that the hearing of most children between the ages of 6 months and 5 years can be tested by utilizing an operant conditioning paradigm with a response task that is appropriate in view of the child's cognitive and motor development.[24] For example, many infants can be evaluated by initially pairing the auditory test signal with a blinking light incorporated into an attractive toy (visual reinforcement audiometry). After a few conditioning trials, the infant will turn to look for the lighted toy upon hearing the test signal, usually presented via a loudspeaker. With older preschool children, a conditioning bond often can be established using a game, such as pegs and a peg board (conditioned play audiometry), or edibles, such as sugar-coated cereal dispensed from a feeder box, as used in animal research (tangible reinforcement audiometry). In short, by having a battery of behavioral conditioning techniques available, the pediatric audiologist can choose the approach most appropriate in view of a child's developmental status. As the child matures, more detailed and precise information can be obtained; nevertheless, it is possible to obtain enough information to correctly classify the hearing loss of a young child and, most importantly, to initiate an appropriate educational program for both child and parent.

Once the hearing loss has been diagnosed, attention must shift to exact measures of the child's remaining or residual hearing (i.e., how useful is it?). As a general rule, greater and greater internal distortion of speech occurs as the degree of the hearing loss increases. However, there are exceptions, and measurements of speech understanding — rather than predictions from an analysis of the audiogram — are needed. The past decade has seen significant developments in materials and procedures designed to assess the auditory recognition abilities of preschoolers.[25,26,27,28]

One test, suitable for use with hearing-impaired children ages 4 to 12, is the Test of Auditory Comprehension.[29] This measure consists of 10 auditory subtests scaled in difficulty from recognition of familiar environmental sounds to answering questions after listening to a story in a background of noise. Two features of this test are especially appealing. First, the test has been standardized on a relatively large sample of hearing-impaired children who vary in age and degree of impairment; therefore, the score achieved by a particular child can be compared with that achieved by hearing-impaired peers. Such a comparison is often useful when counseling both parents and teachers who have set unrealistic levels of expectation relative to auditory function. Second, the test is accompanied by a curriculum containing suggestions for auditory activities appropriate for use in either a classroom or resource room. Unlike adults with acquired hearing loss, it is anticipated that in children emerging auditory skills will become apparent with training and maturation. For example, children with mild and moderate degrees of hearing impairment typically learn to discriminate and identify both common environmental sounds and familiar words, phrases, and sentences after being properly fitted with hearing aids. In sharp contrast, the vast majority of youngsters with profound impairments develop limited use of residual hearing, even after years of hearing aid use and auditory stimulation — a finding that many proponents of a strict oral/aural approach continue to ignore or deny. It is a rare child with a profound bilateral loss who can recognize even familiar single words in a normal conversational situation through hearing alone. This statement is confirmed by analysis of the normative data for the Test of Auditory Comprehension relative to the performance of children ages 4 through 12 with profound bilateral losses. With early and consistent training, such children may utilize their residual hearing as an alerting sense and as a means to monitor the loudness and patterning of their own speech.

Hearing-impaired children who deserve special consideration are those with severe impairments (65–85 dB). Such children, in my clinical experience, may function either as primary auditory or primary visual learners, depending on their sensory experiences during the early preschool years. Stated differently, they may function as either hard-of-hearing or deaf.

Although the preceding discussion has focused heavily upon degree of hearing loss as a primary determinant of a child's level of auditory function, it must be recognized that a host of additional variables interact and ultimately determine each youngster's use of hearing.[30] Certainly, the age of identification, the age a language stimulation program using amplification is initiated, and the quality of the child's experiences in the home are major variables. The presence of additional deficits, including damage to the central auditory system, will impact on the child's auditory, cognitive, and linguistic development. As mentioned earlier, the prevalence of multihandicapped hearing-impaired children has increased as advances in neonatal and pediatric medicine have developed. For this reason, the pure tone audiogram alone can be quite misleading relative to a child's auditory potential.

SELECTION OF AMPLIFICATION

Once a significant bilateral sensorineural hearing impairment is confirmed, it is imperative that the audiologist consider whether or not the child should use a hearing aid. Two major questions should be considered. First, is the degree of hearing loss of sufficient magnitude to result in a developmental language delay? Unfortunately, many physicians and audiologists consider only how an adult with a similar but acquired hearing loss functions without amplification. Adults who have developed a verbal language system and adequate communications skills before the onset of a hearing loss can sometimes get by without a hearing aid, but a similar hearing loss during childhood can be pervasive in its effects on language, cognitive, and social development. One strategy that can highlight the effect of a hearing loss on speech understanding is to plot on an audiogram the key components of conversational speech (see Fig. 3–3). The child's test findings can then be plotted on the same chart. This is a quick way to determine generally whether the hearing impairment will prevent perception of voiceless consonants (s, sh, etc.), voiced consonants (g, r, etc.) or vowels. It readily becomes apparent that even a so-called "mild" hearing loss may prevent a person from hearing many important speech sounds.

The second consideration, and one that is frequently ignored, is whether or not the parents are emotionally ready to accept hearing aid use by their child. The old adage that a hearing loss is an invisible handicap is true only until an individual begins to use amplification. The hearing aid, which becomes the visible indicator of a child's impairment, may result in parental rejection and denial unless the audiologist is sensitive to this issue and prepared either to provide appropriate guidance and counseling or refer to someone who will.

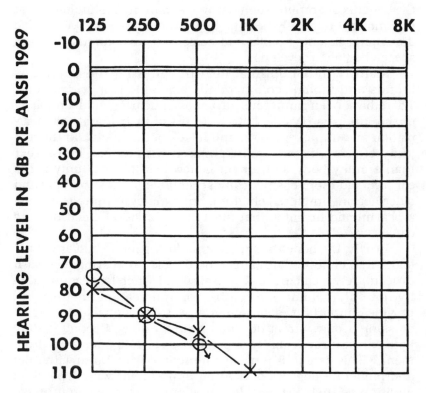

Figure 3–3. *The acoustic spectrum of conversational speech superimposed upon an audiogram. By plotting the unaided and aided responses on this form it is possible to determine which speech sounds are audible.*

If the parents and the audiologist are in agreement to proceed with the selection of a hearing aid, it is critical that a realistic level of expectation of hearing aid use be clearly communicated to the parents. Many parents and, unfortunately, some teachers and clinicians, view the hearing aid as a "new ear." Unlike corrections to most visual impairments, significant limitations in aided listening will be apparent, even with an optimal hearing aid fitting, in group situations and noisy environments. Clinical experience and research has clearly indicated that, in general, the greater the degree of the hearing loss, the more limited the benefits of amplification in terms of speech understanding. Additionally, an extended period of hearing aid use and auditory stimulation is needed with many young children before the benefits of amplification become apparent. (It should be kept in mind that normally hearing infants spend the first year of life developing listening skills and basic receptive language before speech begins to develop.)

Identifying an optimal hearing aid from the numerous brands and models commercially available is a critical step. There have been numerous advances in hearing aid technology during the past decade, both in terms of instrument miniaturization and improvement in amplified-sound quality. In the majority of cases, fitting young children with an ear-level rather than a bulky body instrument is now possible. Not only is the ear-level aid more cosmetically acceptable to most parents and older hearing-impaired children, but a major advantage of such a hearing aid fitting is that most cases binaural aided hearing can be provided.

Briefly, the benefits of a binaural fitting for a child are three-fold. First, children with substantial residual hearing can learn to accurately localize the source of sound. Such localization ability not only enhances receptive communication abilities, but provides important environmental warning signals (e.g., when crossing a busy street or when riding a bike). Second, aiding both ears improves ability to perceive speech in a noisy environment.[31] This benefit is most apparent among children with mild and moderate degrees of hearing impairment who depend on audition as their primary learning and receptive communication channel. Third, the need for preferential seating in the classroom (favoring the aided ear) is no longer imperative when the youngster is provided with two hearing aids rather than one.

Once the audiologist has selected several hearing aids on the basis of past experience and manufacturer specifications, the youngster's performance while wearing the various instruments should be determined in the clinical setting before recommending a purchase. By obtaining an aided audiogram, utilizing the same techniques used during the audiological evaluation, it is possible to determine which hearing aid provides the greatest benefit. It is then possible to further determine which components of a speech message will and will not be audible with that aid.[32]

Such information is of utmost importance in establishing a realistic level of expectation for hearing aid use. In some instances, it becomes apparent that essentially all acoustic elements in speech will be audible to the child while wearing optimal hearing aids. In such cases, enrolling the child in an aural/oral program may be realistic. In sharp contrast, the aided audiogram for many children with profound hearing losses reveals that only a very limited segment of conversational speech can even be detected. In such instances, the level of expectation from hearing aid use must be modified substantially; maximum utilization of the visual modality for language learning and academic instruction is mandatory, as aided hearing will serve only a signal/warning and self-monitoring purpose. For those children with profound hearing impairments who receive very limited benefits from a hearing aid, two alternates to traditional amplification are available. However, both are considered experimental and the potential benefits are being investigated. In one approach, the cochlear implant, electrodes are surgically placed into the inner ear to stimulate existing auditory nerve fibers. The non-invasive alternative is to use a special amplifier to provide vibrotactile rather than auditory input.

Teachers of the hearing impaired should be provided aided as well as unaided audiograms. Also, as discussed below, word recognition scores should be obtained in both quiet and noise. The level of expectation from hearing aid use, and subsequent selection of an educational approach, should include consideration of the child's aided potential. Numerous variables in addition to aided hearing must be considered when decisions regarding educational placement are made. However, in my experience, the child's potential auditory function often receives only cursory consideration in educational programming.

There is growing evidence that the benefits derived from a hearing aid are substantially determined by the acoustic environment in which the instrument is worn. Adult hearing aid users frequently report that their hearing aids are of substantial benefit in a relatively quiet room when they are conversing with only one or two persons. In contrast, they note that the benefits are limited in noisy environments or in large, acoustically untreated areas where there is substantial echoing or reverberation.

Research with hearing-impaired children has revealed that youngsters with sensorineural losses face the same limitations in hearing aid use as adults.[33,34] Many classrooms have little or no acoustic treatment in the form of ceiling tiles, carpeting, or drapes. In such rooms, the youngsters' ability to utilize aided residual hearing is significantly reduced. It is for this reason that many hearing-impaired children use group amplification systems rather than individual hearing aids in the classroom. The most popular such systems utilize radio frequency transmission on an FM channel from teacher to child. The child either substitutes a student receiver for the hearing aid or interfaces the FM receiver with the hearing aid, while the teacher wears a small lavalier microphone-transmitter. This system assures that each youngster receives an audible signal regardless of location in the classroom. By placing the microphone within a few inches of the teacher's mouth, the adverse effects of reverberation and environmental noise are minimized. As increasing numbers of children are mainstreamed into regular classrooms where acoustic treatment is limited, broader use of FM amplification systems in preference to hearing aids should be encouraged.

SUMMARY

This chapter has acquainted the reader with major developments over the past few years in pediatric audiology. It is apparent that substantial improvements in service delivery, as compared to a decade ago, are now possible. Young children at risk for hearing loss should get an audiological evaluation even if their parents have been told that the child will probably outgrow the problem or is too young for hearing testing.

Once a sensorineural hearing loss has been identified and described through a comprehensive audiologic evaluation, the potential benefits of amplification, both personal and in the classroom, should be explored. As more hearing-impaired youngsters are considered for mainstreaming, the importance of utilizing every remnant of residual hearing takes on even greater importance. Children with less-than-profound impairments, if identified early and carefully fitted with hearing aids, do not need to grow in total silence. Unfortunately, stressing the importance of early hearing aid use can act as a covert denial of deafness or a subtle recommendation for placing all children in an aural/oral educational program. Neither message is or should be intended. The appropriate use of residual hearing is an inherent component in all major educational approaches. Whether aided hearing serves as the primary input channel or as a supplement to vision, acceleration of language learning and academic achievement is the long-range goal.

REFERENCES

1. Ross, M. (1982). *Hard of hearing children in regular schools.* Englewood Cliffs, NJ: Prentice-Hall.
2. Mencher, G. T. (1974). *Early identification of hearing loss.* New York: Grune & Stratton.
3. Downs, M. P. (1977). The expanding imperatives of early identification. In F. H. Bess (Ed.), *Childhood deafness.* New York: Grune & Stratton, pp. 95–106.
4. Brookhouser, P. E. (1979). Early recognition of childhood hearing impairment. *Ear, Nose & Throat Journal, 58,* 288–292.
5. Barnet, A. (1965). Biology of sensory deprivation. *Acta Otolaryngologica* (Supp. 206), 210–214.
6. Webster, D., and Webster, M. (1977). Neonatal sound deprivation effects on brain stem auditory nuclei. *Archives of Otolaryngology, 103,* 392–396.
7. Sortini, A. (1959). Importance of individual hearing aids and early therapy for preschool children. *Journal of Speech and Hearing Disorders, 24,* 346–353,
8. Downs, M. P., and Sterrit, G. H. (1964). Identification audiometry for neonates: A preliminary report. *Journal of Auditory Research, 4,* 69–80.
9. Downs, M. P., and Hemenway, W. G. (1969). Report on the hearing screening of 17,000 neonates. *International Audiology, 81,* 72–76.
10. Gerber, S. E., and Mencher, G. T. (1978). *Early diagnosis of hearing loss.* New York: Grune & Stratton, pp. 8–10.
11. Gerber, S. E., and Mencher, G. T. (1978). *Early diagnosis of hearing loss.* New York: Grune & Stratton, p. 15.
12. Fraser, G. R. (1976). Heredity, early identification of hearing loss, and the risk register. In G. T. Mencher (Ed.), *Early identification of hearing loss.* New York: Grune & Stratton, pp. 23–32.
13. Simmons, F. B., McFarland, W. H., and Jones, F. R. (1979). An automated hearing screening technique for infants. *Acta Otolaryngologica, 87,* 1–8.
14. Galambos, R., and Despland, P. (1980). The auditory brainstem response (ABR) evaluates risk factors for hearing loss in the newborn. *Pediatric Research, 14,* 159–163.
15. Fraser, G. R. (1964). Profound childhood deafness. *Journal of Medical Genetics, 1,* 118–151.
16. Malkin, S. F., Freeman, R. D., and Hastings, J. O. (1976). Psychosocial problems of deaf children and their families: A comparative study. *Audiology and Hearing Education, 2,* 21–99.
17. Matkin, N. (1973). Some essential features of a pediatric audiological evaluation. In E. Kampp (Ed.), *Evaluation of hearing handicapped children,* Fifth Danavox Symposium, Ebeltoff, Denmark, pp. 93–114.

18. Sweetow, R. W., and Barrager, D. (1980). Quality of comprehensive audiological care: A survey of parents of hearing-impaired children. *Asha, 22,* 841–847.

19. Gentile, A., and McCarthy, B. (1971–1972). *Additional handicapping conditions among hearing impaired students, United States: 1971–72.* Office of Demographic Studies. D–14:1–14.

20. Howie, V. M., Ploussard, J. G., and Sloyer, J. (1975). The otitis-prone condition. *American Journal of Disabled Children, 129,* 676–679.

21. Zinkus, P. W., and Gottlieb, M. I. (1980). Patterns of perceptual and academic deficits related to early chronic otitis media. *Pediatrics, 66,* 246–252.

22. Stool, S. E., et al. (1981). Otologic care in a school for the deaf. *Otolaryngology — Head and Neck Surgery, 89,* 651–657.

23. Hodgson, W. R. (1980). *Basic audiologic evaluation.* Baltimore: Williams and Wilkins.

24. Matkin, N. D. (1979). The audiological examination of young children at risk. *Ear, Nose and Throat Journal, 58,* 297–302.

25. Finitzo-Hieber, T., Gerling, I. J., Matkin, N. D., and Cherow-Skalka, E. (1980). A sound effects recognition test for the pediatric audiological evaluation. *Ear and Hearing, 1,* 271–276.

26. Katz, D., and Elliott, L. (1978). *Development of a new children's speech discrimination test.* Paper presented at the American Speech and Hearing Association Convention, San Francisco, November.

27. Ling, D., and Ling, A. (1978). *Aural Habilitation,* Washington, D.C.: The Alexander Graham Bell Association for the Deaf.

28. Erber, N. (1980). Use of the auditory numbers test to evaluate speech perception abilities of hearing-impaired children. *Journal of Speech and Hearing Disorders, 45,* 527–532.

29. Office of the Los Angeles County Superintendent of Schools. (1976). *Test of Auditory Comprehension.* Los Angeles: Foreworks.

30. Davis, J. M., and Hardick, E. J. (1981). *Rehabilitative Audiology for Children and Adults.* New York: Wiley & Sons.

31. Ross, M. (1977). Binaural versus monaural hearing aid amplification for hearing impaired individuals. In F. H. Bess (Ed.), *Childhood deafness.* New York: Grune & Stratton, pp. 235–249.

32. Matkin, N. D. (1984). Wearable amplification: A litany of persisting problems. In J. Jerger (Ed.), *Pediatric audiology.* San Diego: College Hill Press, pp. 125–145.

33. Finitzo-Hieber, T., and Tillman, T. W. (1978). Room acoustic effects on monosyllabic word discrimination ability for normal and hearing-impaired children. *Journal of Speech and Hearing Research, 21,* 440–448.

34. Blair, J. C. (1977). Effects of amplification, speechreading, and classroom environment on reception of speech. *Volta Review, 79,* 443–449.

CHAPTER 4

Recent Advances in the Diagnosis of Hearing Loss in Newborns and Infants

Laszlo K. Stein

U ntil a few years ago, physicians for the most part did not alert themselves to the possibility of congenital hearing loss unless the most obvious warning signs — family history of deafness, very low birth weight, hypoxia, meningitis, or maternal illness such as rubella — were present. Even when a risk factor was recognized, testing was rarely ordered, because of the persistent notion that a child had to be at least 3 years of age before hearing could be evaluated. The concerns of parents, which often proved correct, were frequently dismissed and symptoms attributed to inattention or immaturity.

The failure to test for hearing loss during infancy can be blamed on two factors: (1) the frequently cited lack of knowledge among pediatricians and general practitioners about hearing disorders, and (2) the equally important but overlooked fact that no one test existed that could rule out deafness with a level of certainty acceptable to most physicians. Despite the best efforts of parent and professional organizations, awareness lagged in the medical profession about deafness in babies, the need for neonatal hearing screening programs or registry of infants at risk for hearing impairment, and the advances made in improving the accuracy of behavioral tests of hearing. Needed was an objective test acceptable to physicians and, most importantly, one they would feel confident in utilizing with their patients.

Interest in the development of an objective test of hearing for use with infants began in the late 1930s. Among the methods proposed and researched were activation of the sweat glands (the psychogalvanic skin response test or electrodermal audiometry), changes in heart rate (cardiotachometry), and respiratory-pattern changes (respiration audiometry).[1] Electrodermal audiometry received considerable attention during the late 1950s and early 1960s, but is now used only rarely and with adults, primarily where hearing loss is a medicolegal issue. Cardiotachometry is still under study, but has never achieved wide clinical acceptance. Detection of respiration and other bodily changes by electronic sensors is used in connection with specially designed infant cribs and will be discussed in more detail later in this chapter. Although often referred to as objective, these tests are more accurately classed as physiological, because each depends on involuntary bodily response to sound. Also important to emphasize is that the use of the term *objective* with any physiological or electrophysiological test of hearing refers only to the nature and recording of the response, not to variations in procedure or interpretation by the less-than-objective clinician who administers the test.

AUDITORY BRAINSTEM RESPONSE

In the early 1970s, published reports appeared on what is now rapidly being accepted as the method of choice in identifying hearing loss in children.[2,3,4,5,6] Auditory brainstem response (ABR) or, as it is sometimes called, brainstem auditory evoked response (BAER), is an electrophysiological test that records changes in the electrical activity of the brain in response to sound. The brain continually generates electrical activity strong enough to be detected by the familiar electroencephalographic machine (EEG) through electrodes pasted to the scalp. The EEG provides a record of the brain's rhythmic electrical activity that occurs normally, or alterations in that activity (as when, for example, epilepsy is present).

Visual, tactile, and auditory stimulation normally does evoke change in the electrical activity of the brain. Such changes, however, are difficult to detect with regularity on the EEG record because they are momentary and easily obscured by the ongoing electrical activity of the brain. In order to identify these evoked changes, special electronic instrumentation is necessary. The introduction of the averaging computer made it possible through repeated measurements to electronically sum changes in the electrical potential of the brain evoked by sound and to reduce or cancel generally irregular and nearly random background electrical activity. Interpretation of the auditory brainstem response (ABR) record is based on the amount of time required for the generation of electrical discharges in the various auditory structures and areas of the brain following the activation of the eardrum by a test signal.

The only requirement of the infant or child who is being tested is to lie quietly, preferably asleep. A mild sedative (chloralhydrate, for example) may be prescribed to help the more active or fussy infant sleep for the hour or so needed to complete the test. Newborns are frequently tested after feeding, during natural sleep. Although ABR in its present form does not provide a complete picture of hearing for all frequencies, it does reveal whether the infant has a hearing loss in the 1500–4000 Hz frequency range, and the degree of that loss. Hearing in this frequency range is critical for the understanding and subsequent development of speech. Therefore, the detection of hearing loss for these middle and high frequencies by the ABR technique does indicate whether the infant is educationally hearing impaired. Ongoing research in the United States, Europe, and Japan is moving ahead rapidly to further refine the ABR test to produce a more complete picture of hearing at all frequencies.

At present, ABR can identify hearing loss in newborns and infants. Not only is this a remarkable audiological advance, but a psychological one as well, as anyone knows who has witnessed the anxiety of parents awaiting a possible diagnosis of deafness in their infant. Although a relatively simple and nontraumatic procedure for the infant, the complexity of the electronic equipment needed, the technical and interpretive skills required of the examiners, and the need for medical supervision of sedation restricts use of ABR to well-equipped and well-staffed hospital centers.

ABR does not replace the audiologist and the need for conventional audiological testing. Because ABR measures the electrical activity generated by the inner ear and auditory nerve

(VIIIth cranial nerve), and at the same time the electrical activity of the auditory pathways in the brainstem, it has been widely adopted as a test for certain forms of neurologic disorders. With adults, ABR has proved useful in diagnosing multiple sclerosis and brainstem tumors. With infants, particularly very sick premature babies, ABR has helped the pediatrician assess a variety of central nervous system disorders.

In a small proportion of cases, estimated at about 2 percent, an abnormal ABR result may not agree with a finding of normal or near-normal hearing from conventional audiometry.[7] Such cases reinforce the importance of additional audiological testing with every infant or child before final diagnosis. The significance of such paradoxical findings is unclear, but preliminary studies suggest that although deafness per se may not be the major problem, some form of auditory perceptual dysfunction may be present.

More frequent is the finding of normal ABR and no observable response by the child to sound. In a study conducted using ABR to test severely developmentally delayed children suspected to be both deaf and blind, more than 40 percent of these children were not deaf as we normally define that term, in spite of the fact that they behaved as though they were deaf.[8]

When ABR was first proposed as a clinical test of hearing, the hope was that it could be easily applied as a simple and efficient test to screen all newborns for the presence of hearing loss.[2] It quickly became apparent that to use ABR or any automated screening test in a newborn nursery would not be economically feasible. Approximately 1,000 newborns would be screened to find one hearing-impaired infant — a tremendous effort in terms of time and cost. More promising was the idea to use ABR or automated screening procedures in an NICU (sometimes referred to as special care or premature nurseries). Known factors that make infants at higher risk for hearing impairment, such as prematurity, low birth weight, intrauterine infection, difficult birth, and breathing problems, are very common among babies that must be placed in or transferred to an NICU in order to survive. Screening these infants would undoubtedly yield a higher number of failures, and might therefore warrant the time and money involved. The combined findings of several recent studies indicates that 15 to 20 percent of all NICU babies will fail ABR screening at a fairly faint hearing level and that 5 to 20 percent will have some degree of hearing loss, but that only 2 to 4 percent on 3 to 6 month follow-up will have irreversible and severe hearing impairment in both ears.[9,10,11]

The 15 to 20 percent initial failure rate is probably due to neurologic immaturity and the higher incidence of transitory middle ear problems among NICU infants. Follow-up testing after discharge to home eventually results in the diagnosis of severe hearing impairment in approximately 1 in 50 NICU babies. The relatively large number of NICU babies who fail the initial screening for reasons other than permanent hearing loss raises questions on the cost-effectiveness of mass screening in the NICU — unfortunately, an issue that may outweigh professional and humanitarian factors.[8]

CRIB-O-GRAM

In addition to ABR, an automated hearing screening procedure using sensors to record the movements of the infant in response to loud sounds has been developed.[12,13,14] The Crib-O-Gram and the Auditory Response Cradle both utilize sensors incorporated within a crib or molded bed. These sensors automatically record head movements, startles, respiration changes, or other bodily movements when a loud sound is presented to the infant. Microprocessor technology has replaced the subjective examiner in deciding whether the infant's response or lack of response is correlated with the calibrated sound. These devices have been proposed as screening units capable of automatically recording a pass or fail decision in large numbers of infants with a minimum of examiner involvement. Extensive clinical trials have been done, but long-term experience with these units is lacking. The need to repeat the automated screen or use ABR to confirm a failure raises the familiar question of cost- and time-effectiveness.

SUMMARY

Advances in pediatric audiology now make it possible to identify hearing impairment in newborns and infants with a level of accuracy previously thought unattainable. ABR has had a major impact on the early identification of hearing loss in newborns and infants. Properly used as a screening or identification test, ABR serves as a first step in the diagnostic process. It does not, however, negate the need for careful follow-up audiological testing and parent–child programming, counseling, and education.

REFERENCES

1. Bradford, L. (Ed.) (1975). *Physiologic measures of the audio-vestibular system.* New York: Academic Press.
2. Hecox, K., and Galambos, R. (1974). Brainstem responses in human infants and adults. *Archives of Otolaryngology, 99,* 30–33.
3. Jewett, D., and Williston, J. (1971). Auditory evoked far field averaged from the scalp of humans. *Brain, 194,* 681–696.
4. Schulman-Galambos, C., and Galambos, R. (1975). Brainstem auditory evoked responses in premature infants. *Journal of Speech and Hearing Research, 18,* 456–465.
5. Sohmer, H., and Feinmesser, M. (1967). Cochlear action potentials recorded from the external ear in man. *Annals of Otolaryngology, 76,* 427–435.
6. Stein, L. An electrophysiological test of infant hearing. (1976). *American Annals of the Deaf, 121,* 322–326.
7. Kraus, N., Ozdamar, O., Stein, L., and Reed, N. (1984). Absent auditory brainstem response: Peripheral hearing loss or brainstem dysfunction? *Laryngoscope, 94,* 400–406.
8. Stein, L., Ozdamar, O., and Schnabel, M. (1981). Auditory brainstem responses (ABR) with suspected deaf-blind children. *Ear and Hearing, 2,* 30–40.
9. Despland, P., and Galambos, R. (1980). The auditory brainstem response (ABR) is a useful diagnostic tool in the infant intensive care unit. *Pediatric Research, 14,* 154.
10. Galambos, R., Hicks, G., and Wilson, M. (1982). Hearing loss on graduates of a tertiary care nursery. *Ear and Hearing, 3,* 87.
11. Stein, L., Ozdamar, O., Kraus, N., and Paton, J. (1982). Follow-up of infants screened by auditory brainstem response in the neonatal intensive care unit. *Journal of Pediatrics, 103,* 447–453.
12. Bennett, M., and Wade, H. (1981, September). Computerized hearing test for neonates. *Hearing Aid Journal,* 52–53.
13. Shepard, N. (1983). Newborn hearing screening using the Linco-Bennett Auditory Response Cradle: A pilot study. *Ear and Hearing, 4,* 5–10.
14. Simmons, F., McFarland, W., and Jones, F. (1979). An automated hearing screening technique for newborns. *Acta Otolaryngologica, 87,* 1–8.

CHAPTER 5

Emotional Illness and the Deaf

Barbara Rayson

I n this chapter I will discuss the vulnerabilities of prelingually deafened persons to mental illness and describe related stresses and mental illnesses, with illustrative clinical vignettes. The deaf share these stresses: their hearing loss always compromises communication, and they live in unremitting uncertainty in their knowledge of the world. Throughout life they must make extra efforts to understand events understood effortlessly by the hearing. These stresses are compounded by the hearing majority's vague knowledge of what it means to live life as a deaf person.

The social, educational, and emotional problems of deaf persons need to be intelligently addressed by their families and the community at large. To distinguish between behaviors indicative of emotional disturbance and normal reactions to hearing impairment may require the assistance of specially trained mental health professionals. Through careful evaluation of deaf children in whom emotional functioning has deteriorated they may discover additional stress factors increasing vulnerability to mental illness. Some of these are (1) traumatic occurrences within the family that are insufficiently explained, such as mourning reactions causing serious disruptions to daily life or a parent's sudden change of mood when threatened with job loss, (2) sensory, neurological, or other physical damage, including attention deficit disorders (the syndrome formerly referred to as *minimal brain damage*), visual problems, and cerebral palsy and (3) a genetic or chemical predisposition to mental illness (discovered through history taking).

STUDIES ON MENTAL ILLNESS
IN DEAF PEOPLE

Given that 1 in 10 persons in the United States will at one time or another need mental health services, it follows that a population with serious communication handicaps will be at even greater risk for developing mental illness. Though Altschuler and Sarlin found no supporting evidence that schizophrenia occurred with greater frequency among the deaf than among the hearing, they did note special vulnerabilities to developmental disturbance.

> Hampered by his handicap, the deaf child remains relatively fixed and isolated so that imbalanced development results. . . . Rorschach tests confirm that many persons are distinguished by ego rigidity and deficient emotional adaptability, descriptions usually applying to personalities that tend to be vulnerable to breaks in adaptation. In short, the net effect of early hearing loss and sequelae is extremely distressful and is likely to disrupt and distort normal personality development.[1]

John Rainer stated in a 1975 article, "The deaf child, by virtue of his handicap, the illnesses that may cause it, the confused reaction of parents, and the relative absence of early guidance, is particularly prone to develop emotional difficulties."[2]

Hilde Schlesinger, writing in 1977, mentioned the Schlesinger and Meadow study of 1972 that found 11.6 percent of children in a school for deaf children needing psychiatric services, with comparable figures for hearing children of 1.4 percent. Schlesinger quoted other studies on the incidence of emotional disturbance in hearing-impaired children that ranged from a low of 7.9 percent to a high of 41.7 percent. One Canadian study found the incidence of moderate to severe disturbance of deaf children to be above 20 percent.[3]

The Siegel Institute for Communicative Disorders, Michael Reese Hospital, in 1974 conducted a study in Illinois special education districts on hearing-impaired children identified by their teachers as having "emotional/behavioral (E/B) disturbances." Of a total of 1,059 deaf children (ages 5 through 18), 28.3 percent were identified by teachers as having such disturbances. Teachers rated 50 percent of male multihandicapped elementary hearing-impaired students as behaviorally disturbed. This study found overall more E/B disturbance among elementary school deaf students than among deaf high schoolers.[4] Mc-Cay Vernon reported in a 1980 article that "roughly 15 to 25 percent of deaf youth are dropped from school for broadly defined behavioral disorders. These youth need psychiatric and psychological help which they are presently not receiving. As a consequence, they are winding up in penal institutions, state mental hospitals, *etc.*"[5]

Not until the mid-1950s was the first mental health clinic opened to serve hearing-impaired patients. A 1977 report found that 700 to 800 hearing-impaired clients throughout the country were receiving services for emotional disturbance. Experts estimated that 50 times this many deaf persons were in need of, but unable to obtain, mental health services.[6]

Deaf clients have the same range of emotional problems as hearing people, varying from temporary adjustment problems to neurosis, impulse disorders, affective illness (e.g., depression), and schizophrenia. For a long time, however, the services offered to deaf people were largely limited to behavioral management and medication, the assumption being that a "talking therapy" (traditional psychotherapy) was not suitable for people with communication problems. This latter form of therapy is based on the belief that a person can find self-understanding and emotional release through verbally exploring painful and confused feelings and thoughts with a mental health professional. Because, in the past, hearing therapists often did not appreciate the communication richness of sign language, and almost never knew the language, the deaf person lost the chance to develop deeper insight into his or her feelings, and thus better emotional stability. For example, deaf people were deprived of a chance to understand the ways that emotional reactions that were related to childhood experiences and not appropriate to current relationships prevented them from responding in new ways to new challenges.

Recently a number of mental health services for deaf clients have opened in the United States and other countries. Still inadequate in number, these programs offer group and individual treatment ranging from behavior modification programs to indepth psychotherapy. Some innovative work has been done through group therapy sessions offered to deaf students in public high schools.[7] St. Elizabeth's Hospital in Washington, DC, has done pioneering work in psychodrama for the deaf.[8]

TWO CASE STUDIES ON PERSONS AT RISK FOR THE DEVELOPMENT OF EMOTIONAL ILLNESS

Bill

Bill was the oldest of four children and the only deaf member of the family. His parents worked hard to support the family and increasingly turned to alcohol to mask their depression. Bill himself had problems in controlling his temper. He was tall and well built and might have found an outlet for his aggression and at the same time bolstered his self-image through athletics. Tragically, at the age of 10, he was injured in a truck accident and lost his right arm. His parents neither knew sign language, nor were they equipped psychologically to help him cope with the accident. They ignored complaints from school personnel about his increasing rageful outbursts.

When parents do not discuss traumatic occurrences with children, the children, like Bill, have a double burden. First, they are often confused about what has happened and may blame themselves for the accident — however blameless they are — and the subsequent disruption to the family. Second, guilt, fear, and anger that cannot be communicated to an empathic adult remain and fester, often being expressed in aggressive behavior. Even when these feelings seem to have vanished, they remain subliminally, often adversely affecting the person's responses to new situations and new people.

A deaf child within a disturbed family has decreased opportunities for processing distressing experiences outside the family with grandparents, aunts, uncles, siblings, or others because, as well meaning as they may be, they usually lack skills in total communication. The child is left to manage his or her emotional pain alone.

Children who must adjust to an event that has drastically changed their functioning or appearance have a pressing need to talk with empathic adults, to reprocess the experience. They need to mourn. When parents of deaf children cannot communicate with them, or are psychologically incapable of coping effectively with the trauma, whether it is deafness or some other disruptive occurrence within the family, the child remains imprisoned in pain.

In the effort to manage pain, children are in grave danger of developing maladaptive psychological patterns. This is what happened to Bill. By the time he was brought for help, he had become antisocial. The court responded leniently because of his deafness. Bill was receiving inconsistent responses from his home and from society. Ill-advised leniency of parents and the legal system can reinforce the antisocial behavior of troubled deaf children. Bill never developed a sufficiently judicious regard for societal demands, primarily because his childhood needs for empathic understanding and consistent guidance had not been met. He had not learned to modulate his aggression. He could not experience the rewards of satisfying personal relationships that compensate for giving up the need for immediate gratification. Furthermore, Bill's emotional problems had damaged his capacity to learn.

Educational failure and emotional disorders are tangled threads in the fabric of underachievement that plagues many deaf children. Although appropriate and early educational intervention are essential for deaf children, sensitive responses to emotional problems, when they appear, facilitate educational progress.

Bill's behavioral problems had been ignored for a long time. Psychotherapists for deaf children can offer more effective help to parents and children when there is a relatively short time between the onset of symptoms and referral for psychological assessment. There are some differences in normal behavior for deaf and hearing children, but parents and teachers should avoid ignoring a true behavior problem by ascribing it to deafness. A reasonable guide for judging the appropriateness of a deaf child's emotional reactions is to ask if this behavior would be considered indicative of serious disturbance were it to appear in a hearing child.

M.C.

M.C. a tall, elderly, college-educated oral woman, appeared at a local community social agency and threatened to commit suicide if not offered immediate therapy. The woman was extremely unstable emotionally and was in great distress over a recent rejection by an old friend. M.C. had a long history of rapid mood swings between frightening depression and euphoric overexcitability, a condition that probably resulted from a genetic predisposition to manic-depressive illness. The patient traced some of her problems to suddenly and without explanation having been separated from her family and placed in a residential school for the deaf at the age of 5. The trauma over rejection by her friend was a replay of childhood anxiety over separation. However, M.C. had other problems. She was trying to cope with the challenge of advancing years and living on a low income. Friends and relatives were dying. Most significantly, this person had a particularly painful response to the insult of deafness itself. There was a wish to protect self-esteem by demonstrating superior language and speech abilities and philosophical genius.

Many of the problems M.C. grappled with are common to hearing people as well as deaf — an inherited tendency to mental illness; the problems of aging, with its accompanying loss of friends; lack of money; concern about personal capabilities; and the lingering effects of an early separation from parents. But M.C. had an overriding problem. She was a brilliant person whose deafness in combination with emotional problems frustrated full self-actualization. Like many deaf people who have been educated orally, M.C. placed inordinate importance on having intelligible speech. While her speech was remarkably good, it was still deaf speech. She was repeatedly embarrassed and hurt when hearing people failed to understand her. Oral adults often cannot participate in the hearing world because they reject sign language. Some of them form organizations with other oral deaf adults. Others, even the brightest and most verbal, may never be able to work through the insult of deafness to their self-esteem.

M.C. longed for a forum to discuss all that she had read and her mystical insights. She sought constantly to protect herself from experiences that would puncture her fantasies of astounding the world with spiritual understanding in excess of that possessed by anyone who could hear.

This person was suffering from a narcissistic personality disorder. This is an emotional problem characterized by a self-concept vacillating between extreme fantasies of self-importance and convictions of worthlessness, accompanied by the expectation of special attention from others and overpowering anger when criticized or rejected. Persons suffering from such a disorder cannot acquire a comfortable or realistic balance in their view of themselves and so remain exquisitely vulnerable to acceptance or rejection by other people.

Fears that her speech would not be understood often prevented M.C. from attending social gatherings to which she was invited. Group events attended by hearing people are stressful for deaf people, even those who can read lips and respond satisfactorily in one-to-one conversation. For M.C., they posed the special threat of once again experiencing embarrassment over her speech and confusion in the midst of so much conflicting sound.

Perhaps those persons whose natural abilities are more verbal and linguistic than visual-spatial or manipulative experience the insult of deafness with special sensitivity. This pain might be akin to that Beethoven felt when he, the consummate composer, could no longer hear music. For M.C., a thinker, philosopher, and lifelong student, the lack of hearing and lack of sign language meant being cut off from the lectures of professors and from new learning to be gained from easy conversation with other educated people who shared her interests. Most deaf persons with a natural proclivity for language find occupations that utilize their talents, often in teaching or writing. M.C.'s emotional problems prevented her from becoming a teacher, but she did express in letters and diaries her unique pain in being deaf.

EDUCATION AS A FACTOR IN
THE MENTAL HEALTH OF THE DEAF

Just as children in Dickens's time were thought of as small, exploitable adults with no special needs, so early remediation in deafness focused on teaching speech to deaf children in the mistaken belief that this would render them like other children and relieve society of further obligation. Educators failed to recognize the social implications of early profound deafness and the need to tailor a total school environment for deaf children. Greater scientific understanding of the needs of children generally and deaf children specifically, along with a more humane social climate, has produced, over time, changing responses to various groups of deaf persons. Three groups with special needs will be discussed.

Undereducated Deaf Adults

Young deaf adults with little or no formal education are often still in the custody of families seeking improved social adaptation and vocational training for them. More than likely they are part of minority groups. Many such adults, although now psychosocially retarded, once had good learning potential and normal intelligence. Homemade signs, a few formal signs, and impoverished speech comprise their communication repertory. They may possess a few minor skills such as fixing simple machinery or preparing basic foods.

These adults are cut off from in-depth normal social participation with both deaf and hearing people by virtue of their limited skills. Their potential has been compromised by the overprotection or neglect of well-meaning and loving, but uninformed, parents.

Some parents of adults now in their late twenties or thirties experienced their child's deafness as a curse from God or a stigma. In shame over the deafness or fears for safety, they sequestered the child at home for years, keeping him or her protected, naive, and illiterate. Some children remained at home after parents had unsuccessfully tried for placements in appropriate classrooms. Herein lies the second part of the tragedy.

Local educational systems have repeatedly chosen to close their eyes to the special needs of the deaf children in their midsts. Some children were, and still are, placed in regular classrooms with little or no support services. They failed miserably and many left school soon after placement. Others were denied entrance to school, or their parents were promised appropriate services "later" and were never again contacted. Truancies may never have been investigated. This nationwide neglect is a sorry chapter in the history of handicapped children.

Even more neglected are deaf and moderately to severely retarded adults who have suffered from undiagnosed mental illness. Often maintained at home and causing inordinate psychological stress for their families, these adults are more likely to have never had educational intervention or to have had it for a few months or a year or two in an entire lifetime. If school systems were unable to provide for normal deaf students, they were completely unable to educate deaf children with dual handicaps. To this day mentally ill deaf children lack appropriate educational services.

Today deaf children typically attend total communication classes in day schools. Despite the inconvenience of riding a school bus 2 or more hours daily, these youngsters can be educated while living at home with their families. This was not possible in earlier times. Deaf persons now 30 years or older who have obtained appropriate educations generally attended state residential schools as children. Although they benefitted academically, they missed out on the emotional richness of family life.

Many of these residentially educated adults function well in society. A few, however, were traumatized and still bear the scars of having been placed at an early age in a residential school for the deaf without explanation because the family had no means of communicating with them. Some experienced damage to their self-esteem, having interpreted their being sent away to school as evidence that their parents were ashamed of them. They are still angry and depressed over the perceived abandonment. A person well may understand the educational benefit obtained from the parents' decision to send him or her away for schooling and yet continue to feel profoundly unloved and unwanted. The belief that parents lacked caring and understanding has been reinforced by the inability of the parents and child to communicate over the years. Quite often, to protect themselves from reexperiencing the pain of the rupture in their family relationship, these persons, after leaving residential school, separate from their families and develop a social life solely within the deaf community. Alternatively, a few people live their lives as loners, avoiding close relationships.

Rubella-Deafened Adolescents

Another large group with emotional problems are those whose deafness is due to prenatal maternal rubella. Many were

deafened in the 1963 to 1965 epidemic. These persons frequently have first or second grade reading levels, serious learning disabilities, poor sign language, and histories of delinquent
behavior.

Chess and Fernandez compared 171 rubella-deafened adolescents with 34 normal controls.[9] The deaf children were assessed for the incidence of the additional handicapping conditions of blindness, cerebral palsy, and mental retardation. They
were carefully evaluated on four personality characteristics often reported to be associated with deafness: hyperactivity, impulsivity, rigidity, and suspiciousness. These researchers noted
that only 25 percent of deaf rubella adolescents with no other
handicaps exhibited any of these personality characteristics
(usually impulsivity), whereas 68 percent of the deaf multihandicapped students exhibited them.

The researchers found the incidence of suspiciousness to be
insignificant in both populations, but found significant differences in hyperactivity, impulsivity, and rigidity between children whose only handicap was deafness and those who had
multiple handicaps. They concluded that the constellation of behavior symptoms often considered as characteristic of deaf children in general should be attributed only to deaf children who
are multihandicapped due to rubella. Such children often have
poor self-control and impaired social behaviors including
stronger tendencies toward self-abusive behaviors. Thus when a
deaf child has an impulse disorder, makes poor educational progress, has low frustration tolerance, and has problems in maintaining focused attention, these difficulties usually stem from
additional neurological dysfunction, not the hearing loss.

Learning disabilities and attention deficits are seen in
youngsters whose deafness has come from diseases other than
rubella. Mindel, Vernon, Rainer and others have stressed the importance of recognizing the impact of neurological disorders
upon behavior of the deaf.

The most seriously educationally and socially handicapped
of the rubella adolescents often come from disadvantaged
homes in which they are one of many children, yet hardly an integral part of the family because no one in the family knows sign
language. Frequently the recipients of an oral education that did
not meet their needs, these students attended area schools and
lived at home. Their parents received little education about their
children's deafness and were baffled by their behavior problems.

In late grade school, many of these students were exposed for the first time to a newly adopted program — total communication. By this time the combination of inappropriate language education and failure to redress their learning disabilities and emotional problems, compounded by lack of communication within the family, had taken their toll. There was then little likelihood of acquiring needed communication, basic education, and an integrated sense of self. A few of these adolescents responded to their special deficiencies and vulnerabilities with psychosis. Some others exhibited uncontrolled aggressivity and antisocial acting-out. Such behaviors create a smoke screen, masking humiliating educational failure, lack of social skills, loneliness, depression, and despair. Persons with this history are at risk for alcohol and/or substance abuse as they confront their inability to find and/or keep jobs. These students are as much victims of societal mismanagement and neglect as of rubella. Although today the sequelae of rubella are widely recognized, there is still no consensus on an effective program of educational and therapeutic remediation.

Deaf Infants

A third generation of children, between a few months and 3 years of age, are now appearing in preschool parent–infant programs. These children, whose deafness can be traced to a variety of causes, enjoy prospects for educational success and good mental health that are enhanced because of early intervention. This includes expert total communication education for parents and children, modeling appropriate parenting of handicapped children in nursery groups, and individual and group counseling.

Stein and Jabaley stress the importance for parents of the opportunity for individual and group counseling at the time of the diagnosis of deafness in their child.[10] They state that if parents receive only "educational guidance," they may develop unrealistic hopes and never work through very painful emotions. Unresolved feelings can interfere with the parent–child relationship and endanger marriages. More parent–infant programs are opening, yet many people still have no counseling offered them in the early stages of the diagnostic period. They struggle alone with their shock, helplessness, anger, and guilt (see Chapter 2).

The effectiveness of comprehensive early intervention as a preventive measure can only be accurately assessed at a later time. We do note that parents of deaf children who have participated in parent–infant nursery programs are more interested in joining parent groups for grade-school children, are more sensitive to emotional problems that may arise as their children grow older, and are more prompt in seeking appropriate intervention. These families have come to see a mental health clinic as a helping place and not a place for crazy people. Nevertheless, there is a continuing concern about the long-range effectiveness of early intervention if parent counseling and sign language instruction are discontinued upon entry into public school. Not only is preschool parent–infant education often unavailable to families for children 3 years and under, but also rarely are these supportive services offered by the school once a child has passed the age of 3 years.

The children now in parent–infant programs range from those whose only handicap is deafness to others who have survived the ravages of early meningitis or viral illness, a difficult birth, or prematurity, and may have several handicaps. These multihandicapped children once might have died, but now live and present complex problems requiring interventions that must address communication, learning, neurological, physical, and emotional problems.

In a developmental nursery for deaf children, multihandicapped children can often be identified early and appropriate intervention begun. This early intervention improves prospects for better educational and psychological development. Considering the obvious advantages of comprehensive preschool programs, it becomes increasingly evident that similar counseling and communication services should be offered to families of school-age children.

AGE-SPECIFIC ISSUES IN THE
DEVELOPMENT OF THE DEAF

Childhood

The normal stresses of growing up are exaggerated in deaf children. Like all children, deaf children face new challenges at each developmental stage, but the communication delay imposed by deafness often has prevented full mastery of expected accomplishments of an earlier stage. Language is delayed; reading is delayed; social skills are slower to develop; self-esteem is vulnerable. In addition the whole family feels threatened, compromised, and pressured when one member is prelingually dead. There is so much to do to compensate for the disability and so little certainty of what ought to be done. Few families readily understand the special accommodations needed by deaf children.

Because of the massive psychological insult imposed by deafness, deaf children and their families are especially vulnerable to the consequences of husband–wife and parent–child conflict. The behavior of children can reflect family conflict. Husband and wife may strive to gain control over such matters as allocation of income, closeness or distance from relatives, use of leisure time, or degree of physical or verbal freedom permitted the children. Some parents may be ambivalent about decision making, handling this by repeatedly abdicating their authority to the partner. A child who requests permission from mother is advised to ask father and vice versa. Underlying hostility over other unresolved issues such as sexual incompatibility may cause one parent to defer all decisions to the other and then greet with derision the obvious errors in judgment that occasionally occur.

When parents are in conflict, any request from a child may result in an adult argument overriding concerns for the child's welfare. When a decision is finally made, it may bear little relationship to the real needs of the child or the reasonableness of a request.

Any child growing up in the midst of parental conflict suffers compromised security. A deaf child caught in the middle of an ongoing battle has, by virtue of the communication problem, little hope of redirecting parental attention to personal instead of parental need. He or she feels ignored, misunderstood, and angry and may misbehave to reassert need. The parents may then momentarily unite to focus on the child's misdeeds without understanding the confusion or the reason for the outbursts. Having punished the child, the parents may return to their original argument. Nothing has been solved and the deaf child suffers continued emotional neglect.

Deep-seated parental conflict, whether elicited or only made worse by a child's problems, is painful and bewildering. A child may resort to self-blame for adult arguments. The acting-out may represent an unconscious diversionary activity to bring the family together, even if only through anger at the child.

Just as divorcing parents should reassure their children that they did not cause the separation and are still loved, so parents in conflict should explain their behavior to deaf children so the children will not scapegoat themselves over their parents' battles. Parents engaged in continuing bitter conflict owe it to their children, hearing or deaf, to obtain marital therapy.

Pathological parental conflict and normal husband–wife conflicts exacerbated by communication problems are only two of the problem areas affecting deaf children. Competent parents working well together can become disorganized because irreversible deafness has struck their child. There is no operation, no medicine, no hearing aid that will cure the disability. Both parents feel angry and impotent but often cannot share those feelings. When parents cannot share their pain with each other and come to some resolution, they often handle decisions about the child in a way that reflects the power of deafness to separate and isolate. The mother may be given all the decisions regarding the child while the father assumes all other power. Such a mother may feel abandoned and resentful; the father may feel distanced, overburdened, and alienated from the child. Many families do work together to support all the members as they work through their pain about a child's hearing impairment. Still a strong potential exists for family conflict when control of one's destiny has been so obviously compromised.

A sensitive parent may recognize a child's rigidity and obstinancy as an attempt to reduce the anxiety, confusion, and sense of impotence resulting from the communication problem. Deafness creates imbalance even when feelings it arouses are met directly rather than hidden. Parents of newly diagnosed deaf children are confronted with an irremediable situation for which their dreams and past experiences have not prepared them. The confusion and the pain of the diagnosis of deafness linger. Parents often respond to the deafness in negative ways that do not fit with their conceptions of themselves as competent and mature adults. Some try to manage anxiety and reestablish structure and normality through excessive activity. They become overly restrictive and controlling of their young children. Such parental controls, the adult counterpart of the child's stubbornness and bossiness, increase family conflicts rather than alleviate mourning over the deafness. The communication gap widens.

Sometimes parents become overprotective and rigid through ignorance, panic, or guilt. A healthy deaf child will react to unnatural parental intrusiveness in eating, toilet training, neighborhood exploration, skill learning, and self-assertion with rebellious and challenging behaviors. Then the parent may redouble efforts at controlling the child. The youngster, having developed expectations of having to fight for autonomy with every adult, challenges adult authority in every situation.

Parents managing a toddler of toilet training age may be torn by new anxiety over this deaf baby who demands freedom to explore and may get injured and yet asserts autonomy with a defiant no when led to the potty. Baffled by this 2-year-old tyrant, parents sometimes turn toilet training into a battle. Mindel and Vernon have noted that harsh toilet training at this age can have the effect of making a child fearful of new experiences in general. They note other consequences of parental guilt over discipline:

> A reaction against the need to teach or set limits through punishment may lead them later to over indulgence of the child. The parents may allow the deaf child greater latitude at home than is desirable for his character development. Those things a hearing sibling would be punished for, the deaf child may be "let off" from.[11]

Inconsistent standards for conduct and unpredictable consequences for misbehavior are often more disturbing to a child than consistently overly harsh controls (not to condone the latter). Parents of hearing children are inconsistent and unpredictable, too; however the frustration, guilt, and empathic pain that wash over parents of handicapped children foster even greater inconsistency.

Perhaps a child of 6 or 7 years is allowed to decide the bedtime hour, staying up until exhausted and cross (because parents understand the dark is frightening to their deaf youngster), but never permitted to play outside the fenced backyard (because parents fear for the child's safety). The child is confused and angry as well as tired. He or she wants reasonable independence because of wanting desperately to be like other children.

> Eight-year-old Bobby built huge block towers on the kitchen table. For weeks he karate-chopped them with his forearm or foot and demanded that his parents or his hearing 6-year-old neighbor retrieve them. Although Bobby's parents

quickly, and his friend less rapidly, tired of his one-sided game, Bobby doggedly persisted, playing alone if need be. Finally, after weeks of this play, Bobby announced that he was really very strong and no one could hurt him or his friend. He started to play "Sorry" and catch and gave up his karate demonstrations.

Bobby's parents thought his behavior was destructive and rowdy, not to mention inconvenient. They resented his wild shouts and his demands upon them, were annoyed at his assuming this kind of authority. What Bobby really sought was for his parents to recognize his growing strength and expertise in their admiring glances and comments. Bobby had the same needs to master his environment and develop new skills that all children have. He needed to become increasingly independent of his parents. He wanted them to trust him to ride his bicycle to the park two blocks away. Bobby needed to be assertive in a way that had not been acceptable in his home. Then his hearing friends would understand that although Bobby was deaf and small for his age, smaller than a 6-year-old, he was neither weak nor helpless. Through his repetitive play, this boy worked to integrate a new perception of himself that gave him increased security and freedom.

Deaf children often grow psychologically through nonverbal demonstrations and play before they use language to explain their play. Parents can support this healthy play when they offer their children the appreciative attention they seek. "Watch me, Daddy!" cries the child. Father's joyful watching enhances the child's self-concept and builds emotional health.

When deaf children start to express in sign language things they worry about, parents need to be even more attentive. Children need to experience feedback and responsiveness from significant adults not only to build self-esteem but also to construct a meaningful picture of their world. Deaf children need to ask many questions, have misperceptions cleared up, learn new vocabulary to express feelings, and bask in a parent's rapt attention. In most families parents who acquire facility in total communication and include their deaf children in the day-to-day family communication have happy, healthy children.

Parents sometimes push deaf children too hard because they fear for their futures and are, therefore, especially anxious for them to succeed in school. Total communication not only facilitates parent–child understanding, but enhances learning.

Vernon and Koh reported that early manual communication is more effective than early oral education in enabling children to score better in reading achievement.[12] Among students with IQs over 110, students exposed to early manual communication passed college entrance examinations at a higher rate (82%) than did equally bright students with early oral communication (51%). Because the students in the manual communication group had deaf parents with whom to identify, some researchers feel it was the psychological aspects of the parent–child relationship that were effective in the higher performance in school. In any case, children with better developed language have a head start in reading; children who have good communication with their parents have a head start in life.

Hardworking parents who learn sign language to communicate better with their children and try to broaden their experiences so they will do well in school may ask what responsibility the schools have to promote the psychological health of their children. Harris has made a strong appeal for the development of preventive mental health programs in the schools.[13] He sees the school as the logical place to develop emotional as well as cognitive strengths in the deaf child. Mindel has argued that the classroom has more potential for treating behavioral disorders of deaf children than the less easily available and more expensive office of the professional therapist.

Deaf children do have behavioral problems to a greater extent than hearing children. Meadow in discussing the 1971–72 survey of school-age deaf children with emotional and behavioral problems (part of an annual study of the Office of Demographic Studies of Gallaudet College), stated that teachers rated only 13% of these children as severely disturbed, whereas physicians and psychologists reported 20% as severely disturbed. Meadow noted that since the large number of children evaluated (33,711) were divided among various evaluators, it is not possible to know whether there were real differences in the incidence of disturbance of children assigned to different professional groups for evaluation or whether teachers use different criteria than doctors and psychologists in assessing problems.

In general, teachers are more likely to focus attention on actively disruptive students. This child who roams the classroom, who ignores the teacher's rules, who aggressively attacks other children — or even the child who loses homework and notes to parents and never finishes schoolwork — these children are duly noted. When their provocation becomes great enough, they are referred for psychological evaluation.

On the other hand, a shy child who has no friends, an unhappy child who seldom smiles, or a withdrawn child who seems to be in a world of his or her own may pass from class to class for several years before emotional distress draws attention. Parents need to be alert to the needs of withdrawn children who cause little trouble but may be seriously maladjusted. Their problems can be more serious than those of their more flamboyant classmates who "drive the teacher crazy."

Sometimes deaf children exhibit unusual behaviors that indicate a misreading of the environment, not a behavioral disorder. For example, both parents and teachers note that some experiences of daily life can be particularly confusing to normal deaf children. Differentiating reality from the fantasy exploits they see on television can be hard for children who depend on their sight exclusively. For them "seeing is believing." These children understand religious concepts at best in a very concrete fashion; the devil, angels, heaven, and hell may be as real for the child as grandmother or the ice cream man. And deaf children are slower than their hearing friends to understand the nature of death.

> Nine-year-old Harriet was hard of hearing and very unhappy with herself. She was doing poorly in reading and felt herself to be a failure. One Saturday Harriet acted out a drama in which an angel with wide, white wings appeared to her and offered to whisk her to heaven, where she would be happy ever after. Harriet enacted her own death, the mourning mother and father at the funeral, and her happy life in heaven with the angels.

Harriet needed special help in school to improve her reading. Her family had two tasks: to help Harriet deal with her low self-esteem because of her problems in school and to help her understand death.

Anxious children cling to a variety of fantasies to avoid feelings of inadequacy, anxiety, depression, and fear. Because deaf children have less access to everyday experiences that correct misconceptions, they need help to understand the needs behind their fantasies and to alleviate their dependence upon them.

Deaf children who have emotional problems are baffling to their parents. Loving parents may have no expertise in searching out the roots of strange or dangerous childhood behaviors, but they are quick to feel inadequate and guilty for somehow failing in the guidance of the child. They may not know that learning problems that frustrate the child, or an inherited vulnerability when stressed, or the physical and emotional changes of puberty are creating the emotional disturbance. The parents blame themselves. When they then redouble disciplinary efforts to stamp out strong expression of rage or extreme withdrawal, the situation may become worse.

It is not easy to discriminate those disturbances which occur as a part of the normal growth cycle and are self-limited from those which presage a deeper disruption. In general, emotional problems that invade a wide range of the child's functioning or seriously disturb school progress require professional intervention. A child who can't make friends or is always unhappy needs help. A school counselor can often help, but sometimes a psychologist or psychiatrist must be consulted. Should a child require treatment, the chances for successful therapy are much better if the youngster and the family receive early intervention than if the emotional disorder is untreated until adolescence or later.

Adolescence

Adolescence is for many young people a period of turbulence and rebellion. Lessened preparation for separation from the family and lack of information resulting in greater social naïveté prevent an easy transition from dependent deaf child to self-confident teenager. Many a deaf adolescent tends to submit for a considerable time to parental overprotection and then suddenly to erupt with an "I've got to get out of here!" Then this unsophisticated boy or girl may become involved with alcohol or drugs or premarital sex, just like his hearing counterparts. He or she, however, usually lacks the incidental knowledge and semi-protective devices the hearing young person has absorbed from a broader exposure to peer and adult cultures. Special deficits in handling sexuality may plague these young people and persist into marriage.

Deaf adolescents may exhibit a cultural or familial coping mechanism such as physical attack when they feel threatened by peers or adults perceived as too authoritarian or as insulting. Modulation of reaction is compromised by the narrow range of behaviors developed as possible responses to injury. An aggressive retaliation will appear to hearing people as an incomprehensibly crude or exaggerated reaction to a verbal taunt. The adults do not recognize the insult as an intolerable blow to the adolescent's already compromised self-esteem.

Many hearing-impaired adolescents appear to mature somewhat slowly. Males, particularly, seem to be overpowered by sudden combined surges of sexual and aggressive energies they do not know how to express.

> Cecil was a slim 16-year-old with acne and minimal school success. He attended graphic teenage films and watched rock stars on television. He had not dated, but had a clear-cut, if limited and concrete, conception of male–female sexual behavior. He was strongly attracted to Jennie, a deaf classmate, an attraction of which she was unaware. One day he followed Jennie to the school basement and pulled her over for a kiss. She resisted the unexpected advance, at which point Cecil tore her blouse and grabbed her breast. Jennie's screams and the timely arrival of the football coach prevented further harm. Later Cecil insisted, when questioned in court, that Jennie was only pretending — that all girls behaved like that, but he knew what they really wanted. He had seen it in the movies: when they were forced to have sex, they loved it.

Sometimes, unlike Jennie, high school girls invite sexual advances by their provocative behavior because they lack understanding of male sexuality. Deaf girls have fewer opportunities to acquire such knowledge and may appear to encourage this response when they believe they are only "having fun" and are really seeking affirmation of their feminine attractiveness. These misreadings on the part of both sexes can have dangerous consequences.

Deaf adolescents are vulnerable to sexual put-down and frequently react impulsively to such perceptions, whether or not they are accurate. This sensitivity helps to explain hair-trigger conversion of strong feelings into aggressive behavior despite the perceptions of school personnel who insist the precipitating incident was "nothing really."

Relationships other than boy–girl attachments can cause problems for adolescents. Occasionally a high school girl will become so attached to a female teacher that the anxious teacher will request advice and intervention from the school psychologist or social worker. Early adolescent crushes on same-sex adults who are objects of admiration are a common phase in sexual development and usually no cause for alarm. Deaf adolescents, however, face problems different from those of hearing friends; these may prolong the attachment.

Adella, a 14-year-old, had a crush on Miss Hines. She followed the teacher down the hall and lingered in her room after school. Then she began to resent Miss Hines's attention to other girls in the class. Feeling rejected as the teacher became self-protective and cool, Adella invented nasty rumors about Miss Hines's sexual behavior and wrote cruel notes to classmates. Inquiry revealed Adella was experiencing a particularly intense crush because she was feeling lonely. The family had moved into a new neighborhood at the same time an older deaf sister to whom she was close had married and left home. Adella's mother, who knew no sign language, was increasingly preoccupied with a new grandchild. Adella was desperate for friends. When Miss Hines was encouraged to be friendly but appropriately distant, and especially after Adella made some hearing friends in the new neighborhood, things changed. The crush and the nasty notes abruptly disappeared.

Sometimes parents interpret the cessation of a disturbing behavior as indicating an adolescent's problem has been solved. In this case, although Adella gave Miss Hines no further problem, she had not really lost her angry feelings nor learned more suitable ways to manage feelings of rejection. Unless serious personality problems underlying unacceptable behaviors are understood and addressed, the difficulty persists, to reemerge later in more serious forms. Then the adolescent may require a longer and more complicated therapeutic intervention than would originally have been needed.

An additional problem, exacerbated in deaf adolescents, is appropriate separation from the family. Many teenagers, less disturbed than Cecil and Adella, experience problems in this area. Sometimes they are pulled by maturational imperatives and their notions of the culture's expectations for independence into violent breaks from their families. Wild family melees may erupt as the adolescent disregards family rules and clings to peers. Deaf adolescents particularly often lack a clear set of social norms or behavioral principles, in part because their parents did not communicate well with them as children. Some of the adolescent anger is a resurgence of buried rage at not having had earlier emotional needs met. Such adolescents may appear more seriously disturbed than they actually are. The love–hate relationship between the teenager and his or her angry, frightened parents is a recapitulation of an early childhood struggle. As always, when both parties to the fray are unsure of their positions, the battle rages intensely. The adolescent, like the 2-year-old, screams no when really meaning yes. The parents do battle over trivial issues, losing sight of the important matters.

Parents of an adolescent usually experience reactivated pain over their child's deafness as they confront the teenager's burgeoning sexuality and their own concerns about sexual and vocational prospects. They may alternate between suffocating restrictiveness and unrealistic expectations of maturity.

> Mr. and Mrs. Y felt comfortable in sending their deaf daughter away to college but would not permit her to take the bus to the city alone. Alice had no dates and terrified her parents when she developed a mild crush on the family's minister. Once in college far from home, Alice entered a hasty sexual relationship with her first boyfriend, making no attempt to protect herself from pregnancy. She also was unable to make a rational evaluation of the boy's character or maturity. Her parents, unaware of Alice's emotional neediness and lack of social sophistication, were delighted that she was "normal" after all, now that she had a boyfriend.

The onset of their children's adolescence seems to induce a temporary regression in parents and particularly in parents of deaf children. Parents tend to feel as their deaf children frequently feel — inadequate, helpless, powerless. Anxieties that parents believe they have completely resolved during their children's early years emerge with surprising strength as parents experience the unpredictability and impulsivity of teenagers struggling for independence and self-definition. Parents reenact adolescent longing for separation from the family and fear of this separation in their own ambivalence and inconsistency. Some parents appear to deal with their own fears through overprotection, an unconscious merger with the adolescents' feelings of helplessness. But adolescents only feel fearful and helpless some of the time. At other times they experience themselves as — and may be — very brave and competent. When parents unconsciously identify only with the inadequate side of adolescents and fail to perceive real competence, trouble results. Caring parental love and protection may be summarily rejected. Then parents can become as irrational in their anger and fear as the teenagers may be in bravado and confrontation. Desperate teenagers sometimes are semidelinquent as they grope for autonomy or pseudomaturity to prove their capabilities.

Parental anxiety that insults complex teenagers with a one-sided view results from the parents' confrontation with imagined or actual failures on their part. Adults see adolescence as a last chance to make amends for parenting failures. They need as much help in processing fears about letting handicapped children grow up as they do in adopting reasonable rules and improving communication.

Some parents make the opposite error in handling their adolescents. They may accept a stance of perfect competence at face value and abandon their guiding role. Then adolescents feel unloved and endangered. They may behave in outrageous ways in a desperate attempt to reevoke parental controls.

The relationship between parents and teenagers is complicated in that often the parents are handling the psychological problems of middle age, including the disappointment of career hopes or the onset of menopause. Most families, however, work through these difficult years with reasonable aplomb and maintain loving ties with their adult children — in part a testimony to the powers of love and perseverance. Most parents of adolescents have problems understanding their children at this age, because the adolescents' behavior and thinking are alternatively juvenile and mature. The adolescents suffer the swiftly changing push–pull of striving to be independent and individualistic while wanting and needing the family closeness of early childhood. During this painful but normal separation process, deaf parents often have trouble communicating with their deaf children, just as do hearing parents with their hearing children.

Sometimes an adolescent's problems are too serious to be handled by parents, a perceptive school counselor, or a psychotherapist. Parents may have long since abdicated the effort to communicate with or understand their deaf child and left their problems to the schools, which do not assume this responsibility. When behavior problems erupt, such parents are angry and resentful. They become overly punitive. The attempt to dictate behavior without understanding the particular child is doomed. If parents have never communicated well with their child, there is not much hope, at this late date, for change. A long estrangement from the parents may never be healed. Sometimes therapy will be indicated to help the adolescent resolve excessive anger at the family, low self-esteem, or age-appropriate developmental issues. However, if the adolescent's development is basically solid, most likely he or she can become a well-functioning adult despite the absence of close cognitive interaction with parents.

Sometimes a school counselor can give the adolescent the relationship needed for further growth. Despite poor parent--child communication, an adolescent with good language skills and other assets that build a healthy self-concept (such as social or athletic ability) has a reasonable chance to work out emotional problems either alone or with a good therapist.

Sometimes the eruption of serious antisocial behavior in a deaf adolescent is the manifestation of a psychotic process that has been present, unrecognized and untreated, for a long time. When the school will no longer tolerate the behavior because the once "strange child" is now physically mature and frightening in his or her repeated and perhaps violent acting-out, parents are confronted with a reality they have failed to see or of which they have denied awareness. When the person comes for therapeutic services, a childhood history that includes emotional instability, abnormal behaviors, and serious school difficulties may be obtained. Often an earlier referral for diagnostic evaluation was made without family follow-up. It is unusual for a psychosis* or severe aggressive conduct disorder† to erupt when there has been a childhood history of good adjustment.

Any adolescent (or child) who gets suspended from school, has severe difficulties getting along with family or peers, or often appears withdrawn or profoundly unhappy needs a comprehen-

---

*A psychosis is an illness characterized by inability to separate reality from fantasy; perceptual distortions, delusions, or hallucinations; great difficulty in regulating expression of feelings; and serious defects in self-perception and relationships with others. The person cannot carry on normal activities of his life and requires psychiatric services. [16]

†A severe aggressive conduct disorder is characterized by persistent violence against other people or property, often includes theft, and can occur either in the presence or absence of normal social relationships. The disorder may be the manifestation of a psychotic process or reveal an impulse disorder and long-term weak personality organization. [17]

sive medical-psychological evaluation. This should include careful assessment of general health as well as examination of vision and hearing.

The diagnostic evaluation should include an assessment by a pediatric neurologist, a psychiatric examination, and psychological evaluation including projective tests that explore emotional status and personality organization or disorganization. A thorough family history should be obtained. The evaluation is best obtained in a comprehensive hospital program that has a clinic for deaf children or adults. In such a setting, staff trained in the emotional problems associated with deafness and competent in sign language can provide the valid evaluation the patient needs and deserves. Often such a specialized program is not available locally. Parents then should search out the best comprehensive services they can find and insist upon the use of a registered sign language interpreter during the diagnosis. While the evaluation can be costly, it is essential for adequate understanding of the child's problems and appropriate intervention. Clinics may accept public-aid cards and insurance payments; sometimes schools will pay for the expense of an evaluation they have requested.

Often, following evaluation, a program of family therapy will be advised. Sometimes the recommendation is for separate therapy of both adolescent and parents, or perhaps consultation with parents at frequent intervals is needed. Severe problems require treatment in a residential therapeutic environment.

A standard psychiatric hospitalization is generally of insufficient duration and depth to benefit a mentally ill adolescent. A residential setting in conjunction with a therapeutic school for deaf children is a better answer. Unfortunately, there are few such facilities. A brief reactive psychotic episode can be successfully treated in a conventional short hospital stay if outpatient follow-up is provided by a professional knowledgeable about deafness and sign language. Better yet, this therapist should take an active part in the person's hospital treatment as well. Unfortunately, particularly when the child's family is disorganized and overwhelmed, the hospitalization per se is often the only intervention.

Aside from the small percentage of very disturbed adolescents just discussed, the patients with the most serious need for special help are many of the victims of rubella and other multi-handicapping conditions discussed earlier in this chapter. They need a combination of educational, psychotherapeutic, and medical intervention that often is unavailable. We do not yet know the best means of helping these people. For example, to date, schools have not adequately addressed their learning and behavior problems. For these frustrated adolescents the opportunity to obtain success in adult family life and productive work remains seriously compromised.

Young Adulthood

Just as untreated emotionally ill children become disturbed adolescents, so adolescents in trouble may become mentally ill adults. Sometimes persons with adequate adjustments during the school years become emotionally ill when they face the demands of maturity.

Deaf adults in need of mental health services are a widely varying population. There are no typical normal or emotionally ill deaf adults. Deaf persons who seek professional help may have good communication skills (sign language plus perhaps some speech), may be attending college, or may be working, and yet present in a state of extreme stress or anxiety or perhaps in a severe depression. Adults may be experiencing a traumatic change such as the death of a loved one, divorce, or loss of friends or job. Perhaps they cannot control their angry feelings or can no longer engage in normal activities because of irrational fears or suicidal impulses. Some may turn to drugs, alcohol, or promiscuity to mitigate chronic anxiety. Seriously ill deaf adults may have frightening hallucinations or delusions, lose contact with reality, or lose their ability to manage their lives.

Deaf adults who do seek psychological services for their emotional distress may interpret this as personal failure. They may have a special fear of not being understood on the most basic level of literal communication. They may feel shame about exposing poor English skills. Anxiety about communication is often mixed with unrealistic expectations for rescue by the therapist.

Undergoing diagnosis for emotional stress and accepting psychotherapy is a stress-ridden process for the deaf and the hearing. A strongly felt need for services, persistence, and a supportive family are important components of a successful evaluation and entry into therapy. Some hearing-impaired persons wrongly fear that their acceptance of psychotherapy will mark them as "crazy." On the contrary, ability to carry through an application for mental health services and to make a commitment of time and money on behalf of one's emotional needs indicates strength and a healthy respect for the self.

Deaf adults' feelings about their hearing handicap are crucial components in the evolution of a self-concept. Just as parents of a deaf infant frequently displace their rage and guilt onto medical personnel, so deaf adults may continue to blame their parents, often covertly. "Why did you allow yourself to be sick before I was born?" they may wonder. Another response is to blame one's own weak body for the deafness; a person may dissipate psychological pain over the deafness in hypochondriacal concern over other physical problems. Still another response is to turn anger inward by becoming depressed, chronically functioning in a low-key manner that belies true potential.

Deaf adults may accept the ignorant judgments of hearing people that because they are deaf, they are less able than others. Consequently, they may set their goals too low. But resentments over wasted talents lie deep in the unconscious self. The discrepancy between a person's deepest reality and his or her life's adjustment creates ambivalence, vulnerability to humiliation, and an ongoing state of confusion puzzling to both family and co-workers.

Occasionally deaf adults will use their identity as deaf persons to justify venting their rage at the sensory loss onto others, particularly family members. They may use the defense of "splitting": Deafness becomes part of an evil visited upon them by a hated parent. At other times, the same parent may be seen as an omnipotent provider who is expected to meet totally all the deaf adult's lingering childish needs. They may cling to the hearing loss as part of a "bad" self that offers psychological justification for a chaotic life-style and rage attacks. At other times the lovable "good" self emerges in compliant and agreeable "good child" behaviors. When the split between the experience of the "good self" and the "bad self" is extreme, the person has a mental disorder and requires therapeutic intervention. The hearing loss is merely the vehicle for expressing the emotional disorder.

Any deaf adult who experiences continuing unexplainable emotional distress should consider whether feelings about the deafness are part of the problem. The impassioned declaration, "I hate being deaf" can be a step toward accepting the reality and one's need to mourn the loss of hearing. Counseling or therapy may help deaf persons accept the situation, understand its painful consequences and thus free them to experience life with new zest.

The thoughts and feelings deaf adults share with close friends or therapists reflect not only their attitude toward their hearing loss but the developmental demands they face. The requirements of getting and holding a job, establishing an intimate sexual relationship (probably a marriage), becoming a parent, interacting with parents and siblings who are usually hearing — these are primary in the minds of young deaf and hearing adults.

Because young deaf adults often suffer the painful consequences of poor family communication when growing up, they are more vulnerable than hearing adults to experiencing depression, irritability, and loneliness. They exhibit greater social and sexual naïveté and more frequently have resentful and angry outbursts. Failure to participate in a normal family life will understandably result in convincing deaf adults that they cannot look to family for help and support. Feelings of isolation and emotional abandonment crystallize into lost hope for rewarding relationships with hearing relatives and possibly chronic depression.

Chronic depression wears different masks. Altshuler and Abdullah[18] note the absence of the more common depressive signs (including slowed movements and delusions of guilt) in psychiatrically hospitalized deaf patients and their replacement by agitation, generally normal or higher activity levels, and somatic preoccupations. I have found that in less seriously ill adults, depression is often expressed in chronic irritability and low-level anger. Impulsive rage outbursts, fairly common among deaf patients, are related to feelings of being ignored or denigrated. There is hopelessness about hearing people ever understanding their plight. In contrast, in a hearing person a perception of being put down may cause rumination and then self-doubt and depression.

Like pain over deafness, depression can be hidden behind smiling compliance, retreat from the family, preoccupation with problems at home or work, and angry eruptions. Whether conscious or not, when depression is present, it is persistent and debilitating.

Joe, a 30-year-old machinist, complained of exhaustion. He drove his mother or his teenage sister to work, shopping, or social events 8 to 10 times a week. He was proud of helping his hearing family but constantly tired. Joe could not say no to the many demands on his time because he thought this was the only way to be important and related to his family. He did not perceive that his chronic exhaustion, nervousness, and temper flare-ups with neighbors resulted from depression over his hopeless position in the family and his low self-esteem.

Hearing-impaired men and women are often very lonely. They have diminished opportunities for making friends and meeting potential mates. A high school with special classes for deaf students may have afforded an adolescent with a social life, suddenly lost upon graduation. Particularly if an adolescent has been shy or inept socially, the disappearance of a ready-made social world is devastating. It takes real effort for a deaf adult to maintain contact with friends made in school. Social contacts must be made via TDD or letter or through hearing family members. Because deafness is a low-incidence handicap, friends are widely scattered. There is no school bus, after graduation, to bring deaf friends together from far-flung communities. Friends move away or marry; soon there are none left. A social worker movingly described the persistence with which deaf high school graduates return to visit their teachers for years after they leave school, needing to keep in touch with their emotional "family."

Deaf clubs provide social contacts for some adults in urban areas. For others the clubs are not the answer, nor are such groups available in smaller communities. Common consequences of a deaf person's loss of an important social context are isolation and depression. The intensely lonely adult, living and working with hearing people, may become more and more depressed. It is difficult for hearing people to imagine the depth of loneliness that is the lot of many deaf adults. Sometimes the loneliness precipitates the rapid formation of shallow sexual alliances or hasty marriages. Communication problems related to deafness also plague many otherwise good marriages.

The A's, a young couple, were separated at the time they sought marital therapy. Mrs. A was deaf with no speech but had excellent sign language skills and vocabulary. Mr. A was hard of hearing with speech but a more limited vocabulary. Disparate language and hearing, naive notions about the responsibilities of marriage, and the husband's problem in controlling aggressive impulses were issues in the marriage. They misunderstood each other's motives. Mrs. A insisted

Mr. A should translate movie dialogue into sign language for her, convinced that he was cruelly depriving her of the benefits of his superior hearing ability. Mr. A could not understand most of the dialogue or translate it for his wife. After extensive discussion on the realities of hearing loss and communication capabilities and each partner's feelings about them, the couple could better accept and understand each other's handicap.

Communication problems in marriage reflect communication isolation in childhood. Mr. A, for example, complained that as a child he was never included in dinner table conversation and that even as an adult he was the last to learn of his father's heart trouble. Failure to be part of family discussions is a frequent complaint. Comfort in expressing emotional needs is a difficult skill to acquire in adulthood when there has been no practice in childhood.

The A's were encountering another problem. Both partners lacked dating experience in high school. Each entered marriage with rigid, stereotypic, and unrealistic notions of the roles and responsibilities of the other. Because of their narrow experience, each partner clung doggedly to his or her own opinion with resultant arguments and increasing estrangement.

The A's were an intelligent, highly motivated couple who truly loved each other. They worked hard in their therapy. Nine months after a year of treatment was terminated, occurred an event that had been desired but for which the couple had previously felt unprepared: the birth of their first child.

For deaf couples, social skills, sexual information, practical knowledge, and experience with varying relationships may lag behind physiological maturity. Hearing couples usually acquire a more varied and complex understanding of the demands of marriage because as children they picked up relevant information easily. Unlike deaf children, they overheard many highly interesting parental discussions about such topics as money management, role expectations, and sex.

Deaf and hearing children generally acquire the bulk of their information and misinformation about sexual matters from equally knowledge-deprived peers. The deaf child's common pool of peer knowledge is narrower and frequently distorted. The lower reading level of deaf youth prevents them from acquiring social and sexual knowledge from books. They may depend on television and movies. These provide scant assistance in differentiating normal and acceptable sexual interactions from those that are harmful or bizarre.

Deaf adolescents (both those in residential schools and those living at home), at least until recently, often have been prevented from acquiring dating skills and social-sexual knowledge by overprotective educators and fearful parents. It is no wonder that deaf adults may appear awkward and unloving in their approaches to the opposite sex.

A quite separate problem is the ignorance of the hearing bystander to whom the signs for sexual terms seem overly explicit and crude. In reality, the sexual language of the hearing world is equally blatant, merely auditory rather than visual.

We have considered chronic depression and irritability in deaf adults occasioned by poor family communication and unresolved feelings about the hearing loss. We have also noted the isolation and the deprivation of social-sexual knowledge. Another source of resentment and anger is the one-down position deaf people have at work. Often channeled into dead-end jobs beneath their capacities and seldom promoted, annoyed by low salaries and financial problems, these workers become bitter. Such adults may labor for years at boring, poorly paid jobs before building up the nerve to seek a pay raise or advancement. By the time they assert their rights, their anger has built up a strong head of steam. A rejection may elicit a wild reaction that stuns an employer with its violence and evokes a fearful, punitive response.

Judy, a deaf 28-year-old woman, worked for 7 years on the assembly line in a candy factory, watching hearing fellow workers gain promotions to positions such as foremen. Finally another foremanship opened and Judy applied for it. Without considering her good work record and generally positive relationship with hearing employees, Judy was summarily denied the promotion, probably on the basis of her impairment. Judy went berserk. She slashed the conveyor belt and threw boxes of candy all over the department. Then she threatened her boss with her fist. Judy was promptly fired. She could not understand the boss's reaction. She said, "Sure I got mad — but I worked there seven years. Seven years! How could they fire me?" Judy perseverated in raging at her boss and in her insistence upon being reinstated. The chronic anger seething beneath the surface was now unleashed and invaded all areas of her relationships. Judy had lost the self-esteem that comes from being a good worker, and she needed the job. She began to fight with her mother and sister. Her rehabilitation counselor wanted to put her in a work training program, but Judy would have none of it. All Judy could think about was getting back her old job, something her former employer adamantly refused. Experts in understanding violent people speak of chronic frustration as a prime cause for violence. Judy had been frustrated all along, but now was in a no-win situation. Her future looked bleak, particularly when the psychotherapy that was offered to her seemed to have little impact on her accumulated anger.

Deaf adults are given few skills for negotiating their way through the world of work. They often lack finesse in the subtle maneuvering employed by hearing workers to promote their own interests. Additionally, their handicap makes it difficult to establish themselves as upwardly mobile workers. Employers often overlook the talents of deaf workers. Deaf adults have a keen sense of justice, even if they have a poorly developed repertory of negotiation skills. They may have a paucity of behavioral responses to disappointment and tend to ascribe any disappointment in job advancement to prejudice against their deafness. Although they are frequently right, they are also sometimes wrong. Their one-sided viewpoint makes it hard for an employer to correct the mistakes of a hearing-impaired worker. The reaction to a valid criticism is often outrage (the same outrage a hearing worker feels but wisely contains). Deaf workers may lash out impulsively, later regretting it, but the damage may not be repaired easily. The most serious failure of some deaf workers is the inability to look at a situation from the point of view of the boss. Also, from a life history of not being understood, deaf workers often have little understanding of how their own behaviors appear to other people. This deficiency costs them dearly.

Middle Age and Beyond

Despite the complexities in young adulthood, the average deaf man or woman has an established and often comfortable identity by the time middle age arrives. Proportionately fewer middle-aged adults, for example, refer themselves for psycho-therapy. Those who do seek help are (1) persons with serious family problems, (2) lonely people who have never resolved feelings of inadequacy and may have failed at work or intimate relationships, (3) seriously ill people who have previously required psychiatric services, and (4) adults with progressive or sudden adventitious deafness.

The deaf and hearing confront similar mid-life challenges. Disappointment at failing to achieve adolescent dreams, assisting children in leaving home to make their own lives, accepting physical decline and lessened sexuality, and caring for aged relatives — these are major stresses of middle years.

Some middle-aged adults do require psychological services. A sudden deterioration in managing one's life or in relating to others signals a need for therapeutic intervention. Family members may wonder what caused the person's emotional illness. A particular incident may have precipitated the illness, but frequently the adult has an underlying weakness (physical, mental, or emotional) that has diminished the capacity to handle stress.

As in middle age, elderly deaf and hearing people must cope with the same psychological and philosophical issues. Did I accomplish enough with my life? Who still cares about me? Are my children and grandchildren doing well? Will there be enough money? Will I get a painful illness? How long will I live? Has my life had meaning? What is death like? And the deaf may still wonder, why me rather than another?

Gaylene Becker, in *Growing Old in Silence*,[19] notes that identification with the deaf community is vital among coping strategies of elderly deaf people; they tend to increase their activities in voluntary organizations serving their deaf age group. This contrasts with the social patterns of aged hearing people. Becker suggests that the emphasis by the deaf community on the importance of sociability in contrast to achievement serves elderly deaf people well. We can hypothesize that for them the bond of American Sign Language and a common cultural background continue to serve social cohesiveness. Although aged deaf adults may be better prepared than the aged hearing to cope with isolation, having always lived with a degree of loneliness, they average two to three times as many close friends as the hearing elderly. They may also be more comfortable with their increasing need to depend on other people for help with daily tasks.

Aged adults are prone to depression, sometimes resulting from failure to properly mourn physical and mental decline. Any depressed adult should be carefully checked to diagnose whether the cause is physiological or psychological. Too many medical problems of old people that could be successfully treated are dismissed as the natural consequence of growing old. Depression may have a physical basis.

Some elderly people are vocal in their complaining. Researchers have found that crochety old people live longer. Perhaps their longevity is a testament to their ability to force their families to attend more closely to their physical health as much as to the innate vitality that won't allow them to fade meekly away.

HEALTHY COPING WITH DEAFNESS

How do healthy people handle their stresses? They adopt defenses similar to those hearing people use. Everyone has some weaknesses. Emotionally healthy people accept their weaknesses with equanimity and concentrate on developing their areas of strength. The slow child later becomes a star basketball player. The plain, underdeveloped adolescent pretends she doesn't care about boys and wins a college scholarship. Any sport or hobby that enhances a deaf child's physical or social skill or his self-image is health promoting. Parents need to submerge their protective urges and encourage deaf children to acquire physical skills as bicyclists, swimmers, ball players, gymnasts, and so on.

Deaf children build strong personalities when they have wide opportunities to see, touch, and try; when they are exposed to a variety of new and challenging experiences; and when they are not overprotected. Activities that engage the hands as well as the mind are beneficial. If one takes up carpentry, painting, or knitting, there is a product to proclaim one's accomplishments. Assertiveness is a useful personality trait for a deaf person. A parent's conviction that his or her child is as good as anyone else is a push in the right direction.

Intellectual activity is valuable if a child has a propensity for it. The acquisition of language and the enjoyment of reading better prepare a child for a happy life than a narrow pursuit of speech. These activities are best when they have an outward direction, a focus on a specific topic or interest.

Prolonged rumination over deafness is not healthy behavior. Any deaf child's questions about his or her differences need to be answered. A complaint from a deaf child that he or she has been dismissed by hearing peers requires sympathetic response. Perhaps his or her mother has a suggestion about how to make friends with a rude neighborhood child. Few deaf people need a prolonged process of introspection about their handicap (particularly if the deafness is prelingually acquired) but emotional problems must be dealt with, whether in childhood or adulthood; psychotherapy may be needed. No one should probe into feelings about deafness in a person who is functioning well and who has made a successful accommodation to the disability.

Many deaf people have adopted a healthy form of denial about their hearing loss and its possible deleterious consequences for their lives. The most successful adaptations to a physical impairment are generally made by people who downplay the extent of the problem, demand to be treated like everyone else, and get on with their lives. Many intrepid deaf people have successful lives because they refuse to be defined by their handicap.

Deafness creates real life problems that in combination with other demands of living can engage almost anyone's total energies. The majority of deaf people avoid undue preoccupation with their disability. They treat their hearing impairment as a constantly intruding annoyance for which they must compensate, not a devastating loss. Such people have unconsciously understood that some form of denial is, for them, a very useful psychological defense. Those people who define deafness as a major inconvenience rather than a handicap are using the standard coping mechanism of relabeling to render their problems less overwhelming and more bearable. Whatever their feelings about their own hearing loss, deaf people understandably resent the narrow judgment of a hearing world that too frequently notes only the deafness and its accompanying problems and ignores significant strengths and talents.

Most deaf people enjoy healthy psychological growth, leading vigorous, productive lives. If they ask for psychological services, the problem may be children's behavioral problems at school, family disagreements, or a short-term crisis. Serious emotional problems and mental illness afflict only a minority of deaf or hearing people.

Deaf people need, but do not have, the same mental health services as hearing people. It is social inequity and psychological misunderstanding of hearing impairment that make deafness most disabling. Hearing-impaired people should demand and obtain the respect and specialized mental health services they deserve.

REFERENCES

1. Altshuler, K. Z., and Sarlin, M. B. (1963). Deafness and schizophrenia: A family study. *Family and mental health problems in a deaf population.* New York: Columbia University, New York State Psychiatric Institute, p. 204-205.
2. Rainer, J. D. (1975, September). Severely emotionally handicapped hearing impaired children. *Needs of emotionally disturbed hearing impaired children.* A special study institute sponsored by the Bureau of Physically Handicapped Children, New York State Education Department, Deafness Research and Training Center, New York University, p. 16.
3. Schlesinger, H. (1977). Treatment of the deaf child in the school setting. *Mental Health in Deafness, Experimental Issue No. 1.* Proceedings of the First Orthopsychiatric Workshop on Deafness, Department of Health, Education and Welfare (Publication No. ADM 77–524).
4. Green, B. L., Mislevy, R., Litoff, S. G., and Schleiter, M. K. (in preparation). Nature and relative rates of emotional/behavioral disturbance in hearing impaired school age youth.
5. Vernon, M. (1980). Perspectives on deafness and mental health. *Journal of Rehabilitation of the Deaf, 13* (4), 8, 12.
6. Meadow, K. P., and Trybus, R. J. (1979). Behavioral and emotional problems of deaf children: An overview. In. L. J. Bradford and W. C. Hardy (Eds.), *Hearing and hearing impairment* (p. 401). New York: Grune & Stratton.
7. Litoff, S. G. (1982, October 14). Personal communication.
8. Clayton, L., and Robinson, L. D. (1971, August). Psychodrama with deaf people. *American Annals of the Deaf,* 415–419.
9. Chess, S., and Fernandez, P. (1980). Do deaf children have a typical personality? *Journal of the American Academy of Child Psychiatry, 19,* 654–664.
10. Stein, L. K., and Jabaley, T. (1981). Early identification and parent counseling. In L. K. Stein, E. D. Mindel, and T. Jabaley (Eds.), *Deafness and mental health* (pp. 219–232). New York: Grune & Stratton.
11. Mindel, E., and Vernon, M. (1971). *They grow in silence: The deaf child and his family.* Silver Spring, MD: National Association of the Deaf, p. 45.

12. Vernon, M., and Koh, S. D. (1970). Early manual communication and deaf children's achievement. *American Annuals of the Deaf, 115,* 527–536.

13. Harris, R. I. (1981). Mental health needs and priorities in deaf children and adults: A deaf professional's perspective for the 1980s. In L. K. Stein, E. D. Mindel, and T. Jabaley (Eds.), *Deafness and mental health* (pp. 219–232). New York: Grune & Stratton.

14. Mindel, E. D. (1981). Therapy in the office or classroom? In L. K. Stein, E. D. Mindel, and T. Jabaley (Eds.), *Deafness and mental health* (pp. 79–84). New York: Grune & Stratton.

15. Meadow, K. P. (1981). Studies of behavior problems of deaf children. In L. K. Stein, E. D. Mindel, and T. Jabaley (Eds.), *Deafness and mental health* (p. 10). New York: Grune & Stratton.

16. American Psychiatric Association. (1980). *Diagnostic and statistical manual of mental disorders* (3rd ed.). Washington, DC: Author.

17. American Psychiatric Association. (1980). *Diagnostic and statistical manual of mental disorders* (3rd ed.). Washington, DC: Author.

18. Altshuler, K. Z., and Abdullah, S. (1981). Mental health and the deaf adult. In L. K. Stein, E. D. Mindel, and T. Jabaley (Eds.), *Deafness and mental health* (p. 102). New York: Grune & Stratton.

19. Becker, G. (1980). *Growing old in silence.* Berkeley: University of California Press.

CHAPTER 6

Deaf Parents of Hearing Children

Barbara Rayson

T he birth of a normally hearing child evokes in deaf parents joy mingled with doubts over their abilities to parent the child, fear of rejection by the child because they are deaf, and — at times — envy. In families in which parents and children are all hearing or all deaf, there is a normal distribution of power according to ages, roles, abilities, and experience. Parents in such families have greater power than their children.

About 88 percent of children born to deaf parents are hearing. In these families, there is an imbalance in the usual power relationship because the parents lack one capacity the child possesses — good hearing — and become dependent on the child for interpreting to hearing people.

INTERGENERATIONAL STRUGGLE: WHO IS IN CHARGE OF THE CHILD?

Deaf parents need (as do all first-time parents) help and good advice from loving and tactful grandparents. However, when both sets of grandparents are hearing and the parents are deaf,

103

this support may be absent. Instead of supporting the new parents, grandparents (who may still have unresolved grief over having had a deaf child) may attempt to dominate and control them.

The hearing couple who once felt inadequate and uncertain in raising a deaf child have now become the grandparents of a hearing child and believe they know how that child should be raised. New deaf parents are especially sensitive to criticisms about child management. Hearing grandparents frequently fail to realize that the deaf adult, still their child although now a parent, will experience the same feelings of inadequacy and uncertainty the grandparents once felt as they raised their deaf child. The empathic failure and disparity in parent–child communication are then repeated in another generation.

Deaf parents usually have no role models for raising a hearing child. They may have lacked a comfortable close relationship with parents, perhaps as a result of being away at residential schools. Having missed the best and easiest general education in parenting — the opportunity to model after their own parents — deaf parents may be tentative, vacillating, overly rigid, demanding, or punitive with the hearing child. The hearing grandparents feel confident because the grandchild is like them in the sense that he or she hears and talks. In a pathological situation, the grandparents behave as though their deaf offspring is not merely uncertain but inherently incapable of adequate parenting. Grandparents may attempt to take over the parenting role.

Deaf parents often have to fight with their hearing parents for legitimate control of their hearing children. Intrusive grandparents are not found only in families in which there is deafness; however, the problem seems to occur more frequently when deafness is present, especially if the grandparent–parent relationship was already ambivalent or poor. When a hearing grandchild is born, powerful unconscious feelings of rivalry are rekindled between the generations. The grandparents experience the birth as an opportunity for reparation: for correcting their own former errors in parenting. Grandparents often perceive the hearing baby as the child that rightfully should have been theirs, rather than the deaf child who was theirs. A deaf parent–hearing grandparent tug-of-war over the hearing child, damaging to all parties, can occur. Each generation experiences difficulty in identifying with the one next to it as "like me."

Grandparents are notoriously indulgent with grandchildren. Grandparental "spoiling" generally is not deleterious, and can be a positive factor in a child's life, as long as parents retain their authority and their primacy in the child's upbringing is clearly acknowledged by the grandparents. When grandparents are not only indulgent but also believe — and teach their grandchildren to believe — that the deaf parents are incompetent in the parenting role, the results can be tragic for parents and children. Children in these cases may develop pseudomaturity and an arrogant attitude toward the parents. They may permanently adopt the role of scapegoat, fulfilling their grandparents' view of their misfortune in having deaf parents (a projection of the older generation's buried feelings of bad luck in having a deaf child). The parents' anger and resentment at grandparents and child understandably grow. In attempting to reassert their authority the parents often become preemptive with the child. The intergenerational malfunction spirals in an atmosphere of recrimination and mutual hurt.

PRACTICAL PROBLEMS IN
DEAF PARENTING

Deaf parents may have serious practical problems in raising their hearing children. Not all hearing children willingly and regularly use sign language. A deaf mother complained that she could not understand all that her child told her; she could only lipread some of it. When she would ask her daughter to repeat what she said, the child would become impatient, saying, "Oh, forget it!" and run off with friends.

When friends play in the house, the child's mother understands very little. She may interact only minimally, feeling she is pushed farther and farther into the background by the child. A hearing child of a hearing parent can be equally impatient when a parent doesn't understand the child's communication: The difference is that the hearing parent tends to blame a child's normal impatience as the disruptive factor in the missed communication, whereas the deaf parent and the hearing child too easily blame the deafness for the failed communication. Then the deaf parent feels inadequate.

Frequently, one deaf parent has greater facility in communicating with a hearing child than the other. This parent may become the dominant parent in managing the child. If the father of a young child is the better communicator, a role reversal in parenting particularly distressing for the mother can occur. Her self-esteem based on her perception of herself as a good mother is compromised.

If deaf parents are experiencing marital problems, the disparity in their capacity to communicate with their hearing child, his or her friends, and school personnel can be played out in cruel ways by the more oral parent. This parent may, for example, usurp all communications with school personnel and neglect to inform the partner of the child's progress or problems. The other parent feels increasingly inadequate, isolated, and separated from the child. The difference in the ways partners communicate with the hearing world, a touchy subject in the best of marriages, can become a highly disruptive factor in a troubled relationship. Both parents lose sight of the real source of their problem — their relationship — and focus instead on the misdeeds of their hearing child or blame all their problems on their deafness and their mistreatment at the hands of the hearing world.

Some parents have the opposite problem. They focus on each other all their rage at the difficulties of living in a hearing world. If they could share with each other the pain over their deafness and the real problems it creates, they could work out their problems and spare their hearing offspring undeserved anger.

Deaf parents can be as overprotective of hearing children as hearing parents are of deaf children. Unable to imagine what it is like to be hearing, the parents may believe situations that are anxiety provoking for them are equally dangerous for their child. A school-age child may be prevented from playing with friends a few blocks from home or a teenager refused permission to join the 10 mile bicycle trip his club sponsors. Underlying parental restrictiveness is a core of resentment at the greater freedom of movement the hearing child possesses. The child perceives the parents as unjust, punitive, and hopelessly old-fashioned, and becomes devious or increasingly defiant.

Some adults lack basic parenting information and need empathic counseling in parent effectiveness. New deaf parents, like hearing parents, need affirmation of their capacity to be good parents from people they respect and trust. If this cannot be obtained from the natural source, the proud and loving grandparents, then it must be sought from peers, counselors, or therapists. Deaf parents who have a network of competent deaf friends are fortunate, but this network may not be enough when grandparents are destructive rather than supportive: professional therapeutic intervention may be indicated.

Psychotherapy for deaf parents is often not available, or information about it is lacking. Help may be sought after the child is reflecting in school failure or behavior problems the continued struggle for primary allegiance and control that deaf parents and hearing grandparents have waged since his or her birth.

A hearing child who accepts a subtle, or overt invitation to align more closely with grandparents than deaf parents may feel confused and guilty. If the child acts up in school, the parents hide from themselves their anguish about the child's split allegiance and impose punishment that assuages their guilt. Soon the parents are feeling increasingly bitter and resentful toward their child, particularly if the school problems are seen as evidence of their failure as parents.

COMMUNICATION PATTERNS THAT SEPARATE PARENTS FROM CHILDREN

Problems within the home are frequently played out in communication patterns that further alienate and separate deaf parents and hearing children. Family power struggles may be reflected in the use or rejection of sign language. The dinner hour is a favorite time in both deaf and hearing families for acting out family conflict. One family seen in therapy presented the following situation for discussion.

Herbert and Henry were 8- and 13-year-old hearing sons of a deaf couple who communicated in sign language. Henry, the 13-year-old, was fond of telling somewhat off-color jokes to his younger brother during dinner. Henry did not sign his jokes, so that his parents could understand and share them. Repeatedly the father ordered Henry not to talk at the table and to stop dawdling over his food. In the meantime the parents, rudely ignored, retaliated in kind: They conducted animated and rapid sign language conversations during dinner, excluding both sons and ignoring them other than to admonish them to be quiet and eat. Henry complained, "You should see Dad's food sit there while he's talking with Mom."

The basic elements of mutual disrespect and attempts to gain center stage illustrated in this vignette are fairly common aspects of interaction in dysfunctioning hearing families. In this case, parent–child conflict was intensified because a battle line had been drawn between hearing children and deaf parents. The same pattern of conflict was repeated in most family situations. Henry was rebellious. His mode of shutting his parents out was in part a typically adolescent behavior of (1) keeping parents ignorant of the input from his peer culture and (2) subtly defying their notions of propriety while at the same time using a hostile method of denigrate the feared and needed father, whom he experienced as depreciating him. Henry, like other adolescents, attacked his parents at their most vulnerable point — in this case their deafness. The parents, as in many other families, counterattacked by rendering their pubescent son impotent and insignificant. Henry was not included in adult conversation and was treated, as he bitterly complained, "like a child."

Meanwhile, Herbert tried to gain a foothold in the competition between parents (especially his father) and older brother. Herbert complained that his parents did not take the trouble to teach him sign language as they had his older brother. Herbert was obedient and compliant in the hope of avoiding the anger of his parents and attracting their attention. The frequent danger in families who focus attention on the "bad child" who offers himself as scapegoat is that the "good child" perceives that obedience elicits scant interest. Herbert might eventually choose to compete for the title of "bad boy," if only to redirect parental concern more evenly.

Problems that evoke powerful feelings in the course of conventional family treatment can become explosive when deafness complicates the interaction. Young children need to idealize parents for their own psychological growth. The fact of deafness is intimately involved in parental self-esteem. The authority of deaf parents is repeatedly undermined by a hearing society. Because deaf parents are often made to feel insecure as authority figures for hearing children, they may overreact to normal adolescent rebellion and be unduly threatened by "smart talk" and minor disobedience.

ADOLESCENT BEHAVIORS THAT
STRESS DEAF PARENTS

Anxious deaf parents need to be assured that the rebelliousness of their adolescents, deaf or hearing, is part of a normal (if aggravating) growth process. Adolescents are developing their own identities and beginning to cast aside childhood dependence. Their exaggerated behaviors arise out of uncertainty as they prepare to enter adulthood. Adolescent separation may, however, be more stressful for deaf parents of hearing children because the adolescents enter social communities that typically are closed to deaf people, and thus the separation caused by deafness is widened. Perhaps the movement of hearing children into a different community reawakens buried feelings of being separated and different first experienced by the parents long ago when they matured and entered a deaf community their hearing parents were not part of.

Adolescence tends to be a less stressful developmental stage for families when both parents and children are deaf than when generational divisions are accompanied by differences in hearing status. Deaf families share a common cultural bond of language, custom, and expectation. The adolescents can join their peer groups without guilt and without relinquishing family ties and typically suffer no more than the normal adolescent efforts to establish their individuality. When the hearing world rejects the deaf adolescent or compromises him or her with diminished respect and lowered job opportunities, the adolescent can fall back on a supportive social network. Deaf parents have developed a wealth of know-how about successfully negotiating the challenges of being minority members of a hearing culture. In-group jokes and communication patterns make the hearing world the alien factor and reinforce the strengths of the deaf culture. A common cultural heritage and separate language have been powerful cohesive forces for all minority groups — indeed, numerous studies have indicated that deaf children do better in school and make more effective social adjustments if their parents are deaf also.

Despite the advantages associated with being part of a deaf family, deaf adolescents are subject to the same age-related stresses as are their hearing classmates. Sexual feelings and experimentation, pressure to use drugs, a need for cavalier rejections of family traditions and mores along with uncritical acceptance of peer culture — these issues affect both deaf and hearing adolescents. In any individual case, it is the cohesive parental unit that provides the major source of stability and ego support for children and adolescents.

If a viable communication system is established when a

child is young, parents and adolescent will discover they are friends as well as family when the adolescent becomes an adult. Grandparents will retain their important, but secondary, position as loving and supporting relatives.

CHAPTER 7

Language and the Young Deaf Child

Bonnie E. Litowitz

T he capacity for language with which all children are en-
dowed is present in deaf children as well. For this capacity
to become fully realized, however, the child must be engaged in
continuous interactions with supportive caretakers. The nature
of these joint activities between the child and caretaker have become better understood recently. They are structured routines
or formats in which language is used to establish shared realities and to accomplish mutual goals. Feeding times, bedtimes,
playtimes, and games such as peekaboo or patty cake are the
kinds of contexts in which communication takes place. Language emerges in these communicative contexts as a natural
consequence of the transactions between participants — the
caretaker who knows the language and culture and the child
who is acquiring them.

Bruner[1] notes that the statement, a child acquires a language, really has three senses: (1) the child can create and understand well-formed utterances conforming to the rules of
grammar; (2) the child can refer to the world and communicate

meaningful ideas to others; and (3) the child must be able to use language in an effective way to get things done, to obtain what is needed, to ask questions or make promises, and so forth.

All children are naturally equipped to find the regularities in their language environments out of which the rules of grammar will be created. To accomplish this feat (the first sense above) children only need communicate with adults who are correctly using the language to be learned.

In addition, children are prepared to notice regularities in the world. They quickly understand that there are people, who can be agents engaging in actions on objects; that objects, which exist even when out of sight, have characteristic features and functions; that there are events which follow other events in predictable ways; and more. Interacting with adults who know the culture and language enables children to learn, for example, what objects are culturally important, how to use them appropriately, what these objects are named, and what propositions can be truly stated about them. Linguists and philosophers call this knowledge *semantics,* and it is Bruner's second sense above. His third sense is called *pragmatics,* the uses of language. Pragmatics provides the contexts for the mastery of grammar and semantics, for it is only in order to use language with others to accomplish specific ends that grammatical rules and meanings become relevant.

The interdependence of the child's and the caretaker's contributions to language acquisition is captured well by Bruner:[2]

> Language acquisition "begins" before the child utters his[her] first lexico-grammatical speech. It begins when mother and infant create a predictable format of interaction that can serve as a microcosm for communicating and for constituting a shared reality. [The child] could not achieve [the] prodigies of language acquisition without, at the same time, possessing a unique and predisposing set of language-learning capacities — something akin to what Noam Chomsky has called a Language Acquisition Device, LAD. But the infant's Language Acquisition Device could not function without the aid given by an adult who enters with him into a transactional format. The format, initially under the control of the adult, provides a Language Acquisition Support System, LASS. It frames or structures the input of language and interaction to the child's Language Acquisition Device in a manner to "make the system function". In a word, it is the interaction between LAD and LASS that

makes it possible for the infant to enter the linguistic community — and, at the same time, the culture to which the language gives access.

Like all children, deaf children come to the task of language acquisition prepared to learn a natural language; the environmental support for that learning is critical. All children are engaged from earliest infancy in social activities by adult caretakers, who include them in dialogues as potential participants until the children gradually become full participants. Summing up this position, Kay and Charney[3] observe:

Mothers are merely treating the child as if he were already a full participant in dialogue, and at the same time they are modeling his role for him.... it is a basic aspect of mother–infant nonverbal interaction. The rules seem to be that if an infant gives his mother any behavior which can be interpreted as if he has taken a turn in conversation, it will be; if he does not, she will pretend he has.

Deaf children must be similarly involved with their caretakers for language competence to develop. For them, as for all children, language must be used from early infancy under the guidance of an other (person) in social, functional contexts: to refer to the world, to express feelings, to direct actions, to regulate behavior, to create imaginary worlds, to establish one's own identity, and to be bound to a larger community. (We will return to these functions in more detail below.)

In order to understand current views on the development of language competence and their implications for the language of deaf children, it is important first to appreciate fully the language that deaf children must learn. Therefore, this chapter has been divided into two major parts. The first addresses two questions: What is a natural language? Can nonspoken communication be considered a natural language? It is important to see that one can address issues of language learning without being limited by concerns for specific modality (i.e., we can speak of child language acquisition in general without concern for whether children are speakers or signers).

In this section we will distinguish between language and speech, allowing us to address language without speech, after which we can turn our attention to a discussion of sign language. Because the sign languages used by deaf people seem to many to be different from spoken language, it will be helpful to examine recent research on the status of sign languages and to explore some of the arguments that have prevented sign languages from being viewed as full languages. The first part ends with a discussion of some difficulties that arise from a language learning environment in which the language being acquired by the child differs from that of the hearing parent.

The second part of this chapter describes current approaches to language learning, briefly summarizing the evolution of these views over the past 2 decades. Since 1960 the major shifts in language acquisition research have been from seeking the emerging grammatical structures to categorizing pragmatic functions; from an "insider," child-only view to one characterizing development as "outside-in" with renewed emphasis on caretaker and context. Implications of new approaches for language acquisition in young deaf children conclude the chapter.

LANGUAGE AND SPEECH

Most people wrongly equate speech with language. Speech is the actual vocal utterance that results from air being passed through the mouth and stopped or slowed down by changes in the shape of the mouth or obstructions to the air flow by the teeth or tongue. Speech leaves an acoustic image trace for both the speaker and hearer, and an articulatory trace as well for the speaker. Children use the images they and others produce to shape their spontaneous articulations into speech sounds that match those of their community. The sounds of a particular language are selected out by hearing and speaking children from an infinitely varied sound environment. The child's mind is structured to attend to human speech sounds as it is structured also to attend to human faces.[4] The establishment of early social contact with an adult, necessary for the child's survival, is insured through evolution by precocious abilities in the distance receptors of eye and ear. From early sounds and sights the child acquires language.

Language is an idealized system of units and rules that are used to generate and make sense of our own and others' utterances. Units include sounds, words, and sentences; each combines according to specific syntactic rules. For example, while "e," "a," "i," "o," and "u" are all permissible vowel sounds in English, they cannot combine to form a word, *eaiou*. On the other hand, *hit, boy, a, the, ball* are all permissible words in English but grammatical rules demand that only a limited number of possible combinations will result in English sentences:

The/a boy hit the/a ball or *The/a ball hit the/a boy.*

In the past, linguists took as their task the description of what speakers of a language actually said. Since Chomsky,[5] however, linguists have realized that such a task is impossible. No one finishes learning his language in his lifetime, nor does any one person know all of a given language (e.g., English). Consequently, following Chomsky, linguists took their task to be the description of what an ideal speaker-hearer knows about his language that allows him to create and understand an infinite variety of novel utterances throughout his lifetime. The finite set of grammatical rules that comprises this knowledge is referred to as language competence. In other words, knowledge of a language is an abstract system of rules allowing the production and comprehension of specific utterances.

The emphasis on competence (what one knows) instead of performance (what one does) has not resulted, however, in removing the speech bias from the study of language development. Many still believe that language develops as a result of speech performance that has been internalized; that is, talking to an other out loud becomes talking to oneself quietly. These theorists conclude that without the ability to hear or to use speech, language can never develop.[6] In 1962, however, Lenneberg documented the case of a hearing boy who could not speak (perform) but who could understand others and therefore had language competence.[7] There have been many studies of deaf children who neither hear nor speak but who have acquired language competence. Still, the speech/oral bias continues; and many persist in misinterpreting the human capacity for language competence as necessarily involving speech.

In summary, then, language competence does not mean oral language but refers to any symbolic system that is used by a social group, undergoes change through communicative use by that social group, and is constructed according to specific principles. These specific principles are known to apply to all languages and therefore become the defining characteristics of what is or may be called a language.[8]

AMERICAN SIGN LANGUAGE AS A LANGUAGE

Recent research on American Sign Language has shown that ASL is indeed a language as defined by all properties, with one exception. Unlike oral language, which uses the vocal-auditory channel, ASL is a visual-manual language. That is, visual-motor signs are made by movement of the hands and body with facial expressions rather than by vocal articulation, and visual-motor signs are visually rather than auditorily perceived. Because oral and sign languages process information through different perceptual systems, much current research is concerned with questions of neuropsychological differences that might result from signing versus speaking.

One example of a neuropsychological research question is, Since in most right-handed persons the left hemisphere predominantly processes language, is the right hemisphere of the brain — the part associated with visual-spatial information processing in speaking persons — more involved in visual-manual language competence and/or performance?[9] In other words, is ASL processed by a deaf signer more like speech or like visual imagery?[10] Many researchers are investigating which features of sign language are specific to the visual-motor modality versus which are shared by oral language as well and what the cognitive effects of information processing in a different modality are. Results of present research will have profound effects on educational decisions of the future such as when and how to present reading material to signers. For hearing children, reading requires a mapping of visual images (graphemes or letters) onto previously learned acoustic images (phonemes or sounds). For signers, the mapping may be to visual-motor images, some of which may have included finger-spelled "letters."[11]

ASL has been shown to be a fully established language by all defining criteria except differences in processing channels. It is used by the community of deaf persons, changes over time,[12] can be used in metaphor,[13] humor, and poetry,[14] and is learned by children.[15]

Researchers examining ASL find its structure comparable to oral language. Oral language consists of a small set of distinctive sounds or phonemes that combine according to rules to form words (e.g., "*brown*" or "*blown*" but not "*bnown*") that in turn combine to form sentences according to the culture's rules of grammar. For example, *krk* is perfectly good Slavic but impossible English and *I have my heart in Heidelberg lost (Ich habe mein Herz in Heidelberg verloren)* is appropriate word order for German speakers but awkward for English speakers. In just this way, ASL utilizes a small set of units of hand places, shapes, orientations, and movement (cf: phonemes and morphemes); grammatical rules that combine these units are similar to but not exactly the same as those for oral language.[16]

ASL is but one of several visual-manual sign systems.[17] Controversy currently surrounds comparisons of these systems, with proponents of each extolling its virtues over all others. ASL proponents claim that it is a natural language (i.e., naturally evolving through use by a community of users). Signed Essential English (SEE) or Seeing Exact English (SEE), for example, are systems that use some ASL signs but which modify some combinatory elements to make the visual-manual language conform more closely to spoken English. For example, in these modified systems, English word order sequencing is used and verb endings *ed* or *ing* are added to signs. Such systems may be less free to change through use, except to the degree that spoken English, on which they are based, changes. Some people believe that these are not true natural languages, but are closer to what linguistics call *pidgins*. Pidgins are simplified speech used for communication by people who speak different languages, especially in areas of contact such as trade or markets. Oral English speakers who are not fluent in ASL may adopt a pidginized ASL to communicate with fluent ASL users or may find English-based systems such as SEE easier to learn. However, when SEE or other similarly constructed sign systems are taught to children as their native, first language, the resulting language becomes closer to a *creole*: a language based on two or more languages that serves as the native, primary language of its speakers.[18] Creoles, having once been pidgins, eventually become full-fledged languages undergoing changes that differ from their source languages.[19] Future studies will determine if users of a modified sign system such as SEE, for whom it is their only language, will pass it on to their children and use it for group communication, thus allowing it to change independently of English.[20]

CRITICISMS OF ASL AS A LANGUAGE

Even when sign language is accepted as being structurally comparable to spoken language and thereby formally equivalent, questions remain concerning its adequacy for abstract thought. Criticisms center on two related misconceptions: (1) that sign language is only an elaborated system of gestures, and (2) that visual-manual signs are iconic, directly picturing their referents.

Throughout history, segments of the speaking and hearing population have viewed sign language as a gestural language, inferior to spoken language. From this point of view, preverbal pointing or more general pantomimic actions should be replaced by speech as one becomes more linguistically sophisticated. Any remaining gestures provide secondary support to verbal language, and their use varies from culture to culture: restrained for Scandinavians, elaborated for Mediterraneans. In some cultures excessive gesturing is associated with lower social status and less education.[21] In general, in our culture, excessive use of hands in gestural support of speech is discouraged. Therefore, from this perspective, to be using gestures alone relegates communication to a lower social and developmental level, tying it to concrete situations and referents; that is, only what one can point to and what one can pantomime are available for communication.

Response to this claim is that sign language is not a gestural language based on elaborated pointing. Sign language comes from early gestures only insofar as all language is based on the same common early experiences. Psychologists agree that gestures are important in the development of communication and symbolization. Several researchers have described both the roles gestures play in acquiring the pragmatic competence that supports language learning[22] and the elaboration of a gesture into specific linguistic forms such as *this/that* and *here/there*.[23] Barten[24] has looked at the development of gesture, categorizing gestures by the communicative functions they serve for children: *deictic*, used to point to objects in the environment (e.g., for *this, there*); *instrumental*, used to direct another's actions (e.g., arms raised for *Lift me up*); *expressive*, used to display an emotional state; *enactive*, used to represent actions on or by objects; and *depictive*, used to picture an object (e.g., raised arm and waving fingers to depict a tree and branches). What becomes obvious when one is presented with a beginning taxonomy of gestures such as Barten's is that gestural communication cannot merely be equated with the deictic function of pointing[25] and that early communication by gestures contains the seeds of all the later functions of complete language systems, in whatever medium. (The relationship between early gestures and sign language acquisition in particular will be addressed in the next section.)

Allied to the misconception of ASL as merely gestures is the notion that signs can only represent referents as pictures made by hands in the air. Because one of the defining features of natural languages is that linguistic symbols such as words must be arbitrary in relation to what they signify, this criticism calls into question whether ASL is truly a language; and if so, whether it is one of less semiotic power, incapable of representing abstract or absent referents.

The arbitrariness of the linguistic symbol is evident in the fact that there is nothing in the sound pattern *finger* that would give a hearer who does not know English any hint of the denoted object. Further evidence from other languages supports the arbitrariness of language: in Latvian "finger" is *pirksts,* in French, *droit.* Linguistic symbols are not only arbitrary in their relationship to objects or referents but are conventionally fixed in their meaning by a community of speakers. *Finger* means the object, finger, because all English speakers agree. Speakers do not actively agree, of course; but rather, being born into a language community, they adopt its conventions passed on to them as children from adult users and knowers of the language. Meanings of words are not fixed for all time, but change in the course of communication, through what Rommetveit has called negotiated contracts of shared reality and intersubjectivity.[26] We agree on meanings and then we agree on modifications. For example, *finger* can be a verb meaning to point out or identify, or *Watergate* can be generalized to mean any scandal.

In contrast to the arbitrary nature of spoken language, sign language is mistakenly said to be iconic, meaning that visual-manual signs are not arbitrarily related to what they denote.[27] Even when one can show that ASL, for example, is structurally as complete and complex a language as oral languages (capable of morphological and syntactic distinctions), the stigma of iconicity remains. Examples of signs that have arisen by miming actions on or by objects are offered as evidence of iconicity. For example, some believe the sign for "girl" imitates the tying of a bonnet, or for "coffee," the grinding of coffee beans. The possible iconic origins of some individual signs is intriguing, but there is no evidence that signers are any more aware than speakers of etymological knowledge. In fact, these examples substantiate a general property of all languages: that meanings arise in specific contexts but change over time through use. For example, to use *automobile* we do not need to know that it originally meant "self-propelled."

Those who believe that visual-manual signs are basically iconic hypothesize that early gestures of the enactive (action on/ by objects) and depictive (pictures of objects) types become generalized into the iconic units of sign language. If sign languages were only such gestures, it would lead one to question the ability of signers to refer to abstract and distant referents. Distancing of self from other, of symbol from referent, and of communication from its context are hallmarks of more developed thought or higher intelligence;[28] it is implied that using an iconic sign system would prevent or retard such higher development.

If most or even many signs in ASL were iconically related to what they denote, if they were not in fact arbitrary, we could all be instant sign readers and users. Anyone who has been exposed to ASL or tried to learn it knows this is not the case. Nevertheless, some manual signs seem more iconic than the words of oral languages. There are several possible reasons for this observation. First, many signs used by non-ASL or nonfluent signers are really gestures or conventionalized gestures. These signs spring into use by small groups left by themselves with no other means of communicating, such as hearing adults who speak different languages, young nonsigning deaf children, or even hearing mothers with deaf babies. Sometimes called "esoteric" signing (versus exoteric),[29] these signs have their source in early shared gestural experiences that are similar both for deaf and hearing populations. Second, the units of sign language and the elemental units of pantomime are shared: movements, shapes, and orientations of hands, body, and face. Speakers and hearers who depend upon the vocal-auditory channel for symbolic communication retain a capacity for iconic interpretation of gestures and pantomime; they enlist this capacity to interpret visual-manual signs, naturally looking for iconic connections to give meaning to what they see. Third, oral languages are very old, far removed from whatever their vocal beginnings might have been in cries or natural sounds. In contrast, sign languages, being very young, may be closer to their gestural origins.

A criticism related to that of iconicity is the supposed ideographic nature of sign language. This view claims that each sign, like each character of ideographic writing, is representative of a whole concept. In contrast, each word that represents a concept in oral language is composed of analytic units, that is, sounds, like the analytic units (letters) in our alphabetic writing. Such differences, however, are more apparent than real. All languages refer to concepts,[30] and sign language is no exception. The word or the sign for "tree" stands not for a specific tree but for the concept, the class of all trees, just as the words and signs for "love" or "idea" stand for concepts and not for things. The simultaneous presentation of units in signing may be misperceived or oversimplified by speakers accustomed to hearing vocal units strung out in a temporal or linear sequence.[31] Nevertheless, a speaker is no more aware of the sound units that make up words than a signer is of the features of movement, hand shape, and so forth — the units of signs. Furthermore, evidence from psychological studies shows that signers and speakers both behave in accordance with the unconscious structure of their respective language systems. For example, in investigating slips of the hand (signing errors), Klima & Bellugi[32] found that errors relate to the structure of signs, just as slips of the tongue do for oral language. Signing mistakes differ from correct signs by orientation, movement, position, or hand shape and not by the signer using an alternative aspect of the referent object, as would be the case were signs truly ideographic or iconic. Studies of sign language and memory provide additional evidence for the processing of signs as complexes of analytic features and not as holistic images or iconic representations.[33]

In fact, the supposed iconic nature of sign language turns out to be a naive view.[34] Most so-called iconic signs become iconic only after one knows what they represent. Fears by some educators that signing children will be stuck in the enactive or iconic phrases of representational development, never reaching true symbolic representation,[35] fail to understand that full sign languages are indeed symbolic communication systems. Research bears out this conclusion. Studies of deaf children who have deaf parents (less than 10 percent of all deaf children) as well as studies of deaf children with hearing parents who sign show that fears of deleterious effects of signing are unfounded. It has been shown that these children can outperform deaf children who have not had the use of signing, not only in language areas (reading and writing, although not necessarily speech reading) but also in manipulation of other symbolic media (arithmetic) and in psychosocial adjustment and maturity.[36] In addition, the fear that signing will prevent or retard other language development such as speaking or speech reading is not borne out by research studies.[37]

SIGNING CHILDREN OF SPEAKING PARENTS

All human languages are social. The arbitrary relationship between a symbol and its referent is determined by the social community into which a child is born. Meanings are usually

transmitted by adult caretakers to children as part of their introduction into the cultural group. Language, in whatever modality,
cannot evolve from a person alone but must be what binds that
person to the group. Language mediates activities and interactions with the environment according to meaning shared by
the group.

In his classic description of the developing relationship between thinking and speaking in children, Vygotsky described
limitations in the thinking of deaf children isolated by lack of a
communicational system socially shared with adults. Thought
in these children, Vygotsky claimed, is dominated by "complexes," categories based on concrete and factual rather than abstract and logical bonds:[38] "Deprived of verbal intercourse with
adults and left to determine for themselves what objects to
group under a common name, they form their complexes freely,
and the special characteristics of complex thinking appear in
pure, clean-cut form." Vygotsky continued, "Verbal intercourse
with adults . . . becomes a powerful factor in the development of
the child's concepts . . . and . . . in the intellectual development of
the child."[39] For Soviet theorists, like Vygotsky, it is not important that language involve sound; it is the *"functional use of
signs* [i.e., symbols] . . . The medium is beside the point."[40] Functional uses of symbols include "categorization and classification, the organization of concepts in memory, and the ability to
use language for self-regulation and self-direction."[41]

Verbal mediation as described above occurs first at home in
exchanges between parents and children, then at school between teachers and students. Unlike the majority of parents,
hearing parents of deaf children are faced with an immediate,
conscious decision about which mode and form of language to
use with their child at home. To choose a sign system is not an
easy task for the parent of a deaf child; there are several vari-
eties, and within a particular sign language like ASL regional va-
rieties or dialects exist, as they do in spoken languages. Where
one dialect stops and a different language begins is often as hard
to determine in sign language as it is in oral language. For example, are British and American English dialects of one language;
and how about Welsh or black English? Among sign systems,
Moores[42] distinguishes the "standard" like ASL from the "formal" like Signed English or Manual English and from the "pedagogical" (prescriptive) like Seeing Essential English or Seeing
Exact English. Pedagogical codes are specifically constructed by
educators for use in classroom instruction and kept close to English structure so as to maximize transfer in reading and writing.

If total communication is used, sign systems that most closely resemble oral language are preferred.

If the parent of a deaf child is also deaf, the language of choice is usually ASL. Upon entering school, this child will have to learn either another, pedagogical, sign system or oral language, as pure ASL is not usually used for instruction. ASL may, however, be used informally among students in a residential school, and the child would share ASL with other deaf children and adults. These children become bidialectal or bilingual or adopt multiple codes (depending on whether one views the differences between ASL and English or a pedagogical code as matters of dialect, language, or code). Children who use ASL and another system are like children who speak both standard English and black English, or Spanish and English.

When the parent is not fluent in ASL, some choice must be made as to which sign system (if any) to select. It is difficult for hearing adults to become fluent speakers of ASL. Learning a second language is always more difficult later in life, and ASL is no exception. For that reason, many parents opt for one of the sign systems closely modeled on their native English. These are easier to master because the adult already knows the part based on English and can begin communicating with the child immediately using both sign and speech.[43] This child, entering school, will encounter some form of signed English or oral language.

Some people have objected that pedagogical sign systems are not natural languages, that adults are teaching a communicational system that is not their native language and one that they use imperfectly. The situation, however, might be considered comparable to immigrant parents who insist their children speak the new language that they themselves are just learning. These children often outstrip their parents' knowledge because they deal with other more fluent speakers, adult and child. Most deaf adults use ASL, and children raised with other sign systems would have to learn ASL to communicate fully in the adult deaf community — a community in which the hearing parent can never fully participate.

An obvious function of language already mentioned is to bind speakers together as members of a sociocultural group. Individuals build up a sense of identity through membership in groups. Language, dialects, and even slang express who is in the group and who is an outsider. Primary identifications occur between child and parents. Nondeaf parents, however, may have difficulty in identifying with a deaf, nonverbal child, and the child may experience a sense of alienation from the parents' speaking and hearing culture. Subtle conflicts may occur when a deaf child leaves home to enter the larger deaf community. A recent study describes the alienation experienced by nonfluent signers who enter Gallaudet College.[44]

Nevertheless, in a pluralistic country like America it is not unusual to belong to multiple groups and for speakers to be code switchers, bidialectal, or even bilingual. To encourage deaf children to be part of this tradition is to acknowledge the fact that they, like many other Americans, are part of several subcultures (several, perhaps, within the deaf community alone). To the degree that sign systems or languages overlap, a good foundation in one will make learning others less difficult. Research evidence suggests that multilingualism can increase conscious awareness of language and benefit cognitive achievement if (1) the contexts of different language or dialect use are clear and understood by the child; (2) parents and community share a positive attitude toward both languages; and (3) there is a solid beginning in at least one language. We now turn to these beginnings.

LANGUAGE ACQUISITION

There is no question that the very first years of life (up to age 3 or 5) are especially productive for the acquisition of language. Theorists do not always agree, however, why this is the case. Does language emerge naturally? Does it appear only following prior cognitive (semantic) development? Does it emerge out of communicational contexts?

The answer to all three of these questions is yes. There is a natural endowment that all human babies bring to learning the appropriate forms of language. There is also a way of knowing the world that is uniquely human and expressable by language. These early intellectual achievements are species-specific and determined by the rapid neuroanatomical development of the brain in the first 6 years of life.[45] Sensory handicaps such as in deafness, blindness, or apraxia need not disturb this development, provided the communicational contexts of the child's early years are supportive and nurturing.

Understanding of the multiple aspects of early language development has only emerged in slow stages over the past two and a half decades of child-language study. Studies of deaf children and sign language have provided crucial insights into what it means to acquire or know a language. The earliest steps to our understanding involved syntax, the rules for creating and understanding well-formed utterances. Next, we came to understand semantics, or how children acquire the ability to express meanings. And finally, we have seen that the abilities to combine form and content in language take place in communicational exchanges. Thus, little by little, we learned all three senses (as Bruner notes above) of what it means to say, "A child acquires a language."

Recent advances in child-language research began after 1959, when Chomsky revived the notion of a language faculty in the human brain that enables the accomplishment of rapid, early linguistic acquisition. As a result of Chomsky's work, developmental research of the 1960s focused on the emerging grammars of the young child, discovering how these successive grammars ultimately approximate adult syntax. Comparative studies across languages illustrated how the universal aspects of language were learned first, followed by particular language rules. Much was made at that time of language universals as "hard wiring" of the brain, and of language-specific features as "software." In this theoretical climate, neurological and biological aspects of language acquisition became important. For example, preadolescence was hypothesized as a critical period for language acquisition, based on the lateralization of the two hemispheres of the brain and on early neurological plasticity in recovery of language functioning in traumatic injury. The claim that deaf children begin babbling just as hearing children do, but without benefit of auditory input, indicated an innate, autonomous language acquisition faculty.[46] An active child with innate organization was viewed as making hypotheses about language structure, which were represented in early grammars that the environment either confirmed or disproved.

Early untested claims that deaf babies begin babbling at the same time as hearing babies (but that without feedback it is extinguished in the second half of the first year) have been submitted to careful study. Recent findings[47] have determined that all babies produce precanonical babbling before canonical (i.e., conforming to speech sound formation) syllables. However, while all hearing babies in these studies began canonical babbling by 10 months, the deaf infants did not change to canonical babbling until 18 months or later. In addition, many features of babbling differentiate deaf from hearing babies. The importance of canonical babbling lies in its closeness to universal phonological features, those shared by all natural oral languages. Deaf infants seem to take longer to begin using these features and do not produce the same patterns as hearing infants. Nevertheless, these more detailed studies do not challenge the claim that all children, deaf and hearing, have a natural predisposition to language learning.[48] Such studies do raise further questions about the subtle interplay of neurological endowment, amount and timing of environmental input, and specific modalities.

Even when insufficient input is available, the hardiness of syntactic competence is evident in recent, detailed examinations of signs used by six deaf children (1 year, 5 months to 4 years, 6½ months) who received no specific input from their hearing, nonsigning parents.[49] Goldin-Meadow[50] found the following spontaneous development in one child (2 years, 10 months to 4 years, 10 months): signs for objects, actions, and attributes; ordering of signs into sentences; and combination of ideas into complex sentences. Other forms, such as auxiliary verbs and plural markers, did not develop. Future studies will illustrate the resiliency of a biological predisposition toward language in general and specific linguistic forms in particular.

When language capacity is viewed as innate, needing minimal or no stimulation to emerge or continue, the role of the mother or specificity of environmental influence is minimized as well. In cognitive psychology, Piaget has made similar claims for each child's reconstruction of reality by his or her actions on the world. Although Piaget disagreed with the innateness principle claimed for language, the same absence of specific or adult intervention can be seen in both theories. For Piaget, thought develops from the child's actions. From about 2 years on, it becomes represented by figurative or representational intelligence, including language, by means of the symbolic function.[51] Language itself is not seen by Piaget as a prerequisite to thought. Language merely represents ideas and concepts already formed by the child's adaptation to the real world. The child constructs hypotheses about the world, much as early grammars represent hypotheses about language.

In his early work, Piaget considered language as a mere outer garment for thought. He stressed that thinking arises earlier than and independent of language, during the sensorimotor period (0 to 2 years). Not until the formal operational period (11 to 15 years) is language an aid to thought, although in the preoperational and concrete operational periods (2 to 7 years and 7 to 11 years) it can make thought more facile and enable important social contact. The use of language by children to challenge each other's ideas was considered an important prod to overcoming egocentricity and forcing children to "decenter," or take another point of view. In addition, some social-cultural knowledge can only be transmitted by adults through language.

With his de-emphasis on language, Piaget became a popular theorist for many working with the deaf. Furth,[52] for example, who wished to demonstrate that a lack of verbal language did not necessarily mean an intellectual insufficiency, was drawn to Piaget's theory. On this view, language could always be acquired later without cognitive loss, and difficulties with language were no impediment to conceptualization and problem solving.

More recent Piagetian psycholinguists[53] have incorporated into their developmental theory the American psycholinguistic notion of emerging grammars, which they claim are not innate but rather evolve following, and in order to express, sensorimotor intelligence. While Piagetian and Chomskian theorists may agree on emerging grammars, they disagree on what is innate and ultimately on whether thought can exist without language.

Sensorimotor intelligence, well documented by Piaget and others, is characterized by knowledge that objects, actions, and agents exist and that objects have permanence (i.e., exist as mental representations), even when out of sight. Many psycholinguists have accepted the Piagetian claim that syntax is not innate but rather is acquired on the basis of this prior knowledge. Brown best expresses this approach in *A First Language*,[54] in which he compares applications of several language acquisition theories to available collections of child-language data. He concludes that Piaget's theory best explains the data, and it forms the basis for the first of five stages of language development. These stages are measures of amount of language, not ages; they begin with one or two words and end in complex sentences. The first stage is seen as expressing the cognitive results of the prelingual, sensorimotor period by means of such basic semantic relations or functions as nomination *(that book)*, recurrence *(more milk)*, nonexistence *(all gone)*, location *(sweater chair)*, possession *(mommy sock)*, attribution *(big train)*, or agent-action object relationships *(John eat, eat cookie, John cookie)*.

Second stage utterances are characterized by the addition of 14 morphemes, small meaningful units that modulate meanings. In oral language these are present progressive *(-ing)*, the prepositions *in* and *on*, plural *(-s)*, regular and irregular past tense markers *(-ed, go/went)*, possessives, articles *(the/a)*, regular and irregular third person markers *(-s)*, contractible and uncontractible copula and auxiliary *(he is* or *has* versus *he's)*. In the third stage, basic sentence modalities are expressed: imperatives, interrogatives (both yes/no and wh- questions), and negatives. Fourth and fifth stages are exemplified by more complex, joined sentences — one embedded into the other, as in relative clauses; or compounded, combined with *and* or *but*. These stages have been found in a wide variety of languages, including acquisition of Luo (Kenya), Japanese, Korean, Russian, Hebrew, English, and French.

Research on sign language acquisition indicates that, given the different forms of expression in ASL and English, the same stages appear in early signing.[55] Early signing expresses a prelinguistic intelligence by means of semantic relations; these become modified and elaborated as Brown describes. Hearing and deaf children acquiring oral or sign language move from the expression of basic semantic information to the use of the specific grammatical means in their language to connect longer and more complex utterances.

In summary, theorists following Chomsky and Piaget seem to explain why much of early linguistic and cognitive development spontaneously emerges with little or no environmental input. Piaget and Chomsky both consider a specific environment and a particular adult caretaker as providing only "aliments" (nourishment) or minimal input for an active child constructing for himself or herself a logic and a language that, while specific, share a universal underlying structure. Chomsky thinks the child's ability is innately given, while Piaget is at pains to detail how the child's intelligence builds from innate simple reflexes to complex operations by means of actions on objects in the world; language then expresses this already formed intelligence.

However, sometime in the mid-1970s researchers began to question the narrowness of this approach to language learning. There were two major impetuses to this expanded vision. On the one hand, the theories of Soviet psychologists, followers of Vygotsky, became available in English translation.[56] This work supports the following perspective. While Chomsky may be correct that specific adult input is not necessary for the learning of specific grammatical forms, an adult is critical for the learning of the uses or functions of language; and it is these functional contexts that motivate the learning of forms. Furthermore, and in marked contrast to Piaget, Vygotsky claims that language directly influences thought. On the other hand, detailed studies of videotapes of early mother–child interactions demonstrated that there are pragmatic (i.e., communicational) as well as semantic precursors to language. The combined result of these influences was an emphasis on caretaker-speech, on communicational contexts, and on the functions of language.

Vygotsky is the theorist most associated with the view that specific environments and adults are crucial to early cognitive and linguistic development, and that language influences thought. For Vygotsky, language and thought are social in origin. All psychological functions are first *inter*psychic (held jointly by adult and child) before they become *intra*psychic (learned by the child). Vygotsky and his followers acknowledge a first phase of development in which there is prelinguistic thought and preintelligent speech (compare to Piaget's sensorimotor period). After the age of 2, however, language and thought become inextricably intertwined, with language becoming the major instrument of thinking. Language is also the major instrument of learning; language enables the child to take over for himself or herself the functions that have been performed by or with the mother. Thus, language as a medium of communicational exchange between child and caretaker becomes the instrument for the child's future autonomy, for functions like self-regulation and self-direction. For example, initially the mother directs the child's attention; the child then learns to perform this function for himself or herself. The child uses the same means to perform this function, first pointing and then language. The mother may have pointed and said, "What's that?" The child will point and say "What that?" out loud to himself in egocentric speech until able to perform this function completely internally. For Vygotsky, egocentric speech represents social speech with an other in the process of becoming inner speech for oneself. Deaf children who have been communicating with parents in sign language have also been observed to sign for themselves egocentrically as they take on parental functions for themselves.

In contrast to Piaget, Vygotsky claims that language does not merely represent already formed thought, providing new mental content. Rather, he believes language alters the very processes of thought: memory, attention, all higher mental functioning. On this view, a lack of early communication between mother and child would lead to total cognitive and psychological retardation. A symbolic system, however, would enable the processes of higher mental functioning to progress normally. Rooted in these psychological theories, Soviet psychologists have long considered manual sign systems important for just these reasons.[57]

Soviet psychologists see the first years of life as critical for language learning not due to neuroanatomical maturation but for social reasons. The young dependent child is particularly in need of social interaction to survive; because language plays a special role in that attachment and subsequent separation process, the young child (0 to 3 years) is particularly sensitive to language acquisition.[58]

The role of language in the attachment and separation process is little understood.[59] Nevertheless, many psychoanalytic theorists and others in infant psychiatry agree that the child forms a unit with the primary caretaker out of which he or she ultimately must separate or individuate, and that this process is the basis for the development of a sense of self.[60] Spitz calls this early phase a "predialogue," stressing its communicational aspect, from which develop both a social and psychological self.[61] A critical part of this process seems to involve the use of a symbolic system for internalization of the mother and her functions e.g., the child's use of his or her name for self-reference, later replaced by the pronouns *I* and *you*; the ability of the child to use language to self-soothe and handle separation (e.g., "Mommy coming back"); and the use of negation to test autonomy. At present it seems that these and other aspects of the "interpersonal" and "personal" functions of language are acquired along with all other functions in dialogues with the mother.[62]

Freedman notes that these processes do not require normal hearing. Given access to an appropriate communication system, "congenital deafness does not pose a significant interference to those early processes of attachment and internalization out of which the differentiation of self and the establishment of object relations emerge."[63] A recent study of 17 deaf children of deaf parents did not find evidence of differences in attachment and separation behaviors from children with normal hearing.[64] Such studies contrast with earlier reports of difficulties by deaf children in forming attachments.[65] It seems that communicative competence is the major factor in predicting age appropriate behaviors.[66]

As noted above, the last 10 years has produced a large body of detailed analyses of mother–child interactions. These studies illustrate early patterned predialogues in which are learned rules for turn taking, routines for setting up topics, identification of communicational ends, and means to accomplish those ends.[67] Researchers describe the attunement of infant and mother beginning at birth as entrainment or synchrony that combines sensory, motoric, and affective elements.[68] Some responses are vocal, but many are gestural and involve rhythmic patterns of eye gaze, body movements, and head turning that (along with facial displays of emotions) are equally available to hearing mother–deaf child dyads. Beginning with an inborn attraction to the human face, vision plays a major role in focusing and sustaining joint attention and in establishing reference that underlie such communicational acts as setting up topics and providing comments. Rhythmical and reciprocal body patterns become synchronized in rituals and game playing that are fundamental to conversational turn taking and the segmentation of action sequences.[69] Gestures play an important role in hypothesized sequential stages leading from prelingual to linguistic communication,[70] and retain "important, even if changed and diminished, functions in overall communication throughout life."[71] Gradually, symbolic forms in real dialogues, whether vocal or sign, evolve out of the predialogic experiences.

These studies make clear that communication functions precede linguistic structures, and these structures are acquired as more efficient means of accomplishing similar pragmatic goals: "Neither the syntactic nor the semantic approach to language acquisition takes sufficiently into account what the child is trying to do by communication."[72] Under the general heading of *pragmatics*, developmentalists have expanded their sights to include the functions of language (i.e., how language is used in communicational contexts).

Halliday has posited three major language functions: the ideational, the interpersonal, and the textual. Halliday[73] recorded the beginning language of his son, Nigel, and found seven emerging specific functions:

1. Instrumental: Getting things done with language.
2. Regulatory: Language as a means whereby others
                    exercise control
3. Interactional: Using language in interaction
                    between self and others

4. Personal: Using language to shape the self
5. Heuristic: Using language to create the
                      environment
6. Imaginative: Using language to create a world of
                      one's own making
7. Representational: Using language to inform and
                      communicate with others

No list of functions, however, can be complete, and adult language is always multifunctional. Yet Halliday's functional perspective stresses that the formal structures of language, so much studied by Chomskian linguists, emerge in the process of the child's learning to use language with an other: "Learning language is learning how to mean.[74] What a child does with language tends to determine its structure.... The structures that the child has mastered are direct reflections of the functions that language serves for him."[75] Halliday concluded that "what is common to every use of language is that it is meaningful, contextualized and in the broadest sense social."[76]

The shift in developmental studies from the biological-neurological to the social-psychological has focused attention on how the child's intentionality arises out of shared mother–child activities.[77] In this view, the child and mother are a unit or system in which the child is apprenticed and eventually becomes a full participant. By means of such prototypical activities as games of peekaboo or patty cake, children learn not only the shared rhythms of later dialogues but also how to make their intentions known to another, to refer to the real world, to assert a belief, to request information or demand assistance, and so forth. In language, such intentions are expressed by speech acts which describe to what purposes language can be used.

Although speech acts have their source in earlier, prelinguistic activities, the role of a symbolic system is crucial. Kaye criticized Piaget for "ignoring the dynamics between infant and parents" and thereby failing "to see that parents, as repositories of symbols, are crucial agents in the whole affair."[78]

> The theater of development is not internal. It is an outdoor stage, and the parent is very much the director... The intersubjectivity in the parent's mind keeps a stage ahead of that in the child's, and in this fact lies the secret of cognitive growth in our species.

Parents, caretakers, and other skilled communicators act as if their less-skilled partners are potential communicators in ways that serve both to strengthen that belief and to make it come true.[79] By "arranging" or "scaffolding" interactions ("formats") with children, parents create skilled communicators who know what can be communicated, when (in what contexts), and how.[80]

Investigations into child language continue, with some theorists claiming, "We will have to look primarily at children, not their mothers, to understand language learning," at least until we better articulate a functionalist grammar.[81] Still other researchers conclude, "Although what is learned is strongly determined by characteristics of the learner, it is still the case that whatever these characteristics may prove to be, certain features of the input are better suited to their operation than others."[82] Those features turn out to be amount of adult speech, its use to extend utterances (i.e., picking up and elaborating or adding to meaning that the child has just contributed), and its use to direct behavior.[83] In other words, if mothers are teaching, they are not teaching specific language structures, but rather how to use language to create shared meanings and to get things done.

Clearly, the final chapter in our knowledge of early development has not been written. We will continue to learn more senses of what it means to say "a child acquires a language." Nevertheless, what we already know can serve to inform our understanding of the young deaf child.

THE YOUNG DEAF CHILD

From global beginnings, language patterns and usages become more differentiated. For oral language, many current theorists go back to early gesturing and crying as "protospeech acts" or early precursors to communicational intent.[84] Crying becomes differentiated, joined by cooing; under the guidance of caretakers this turns into babble, out of which speech patterns develop. Pointing seems to play a similar role for sign language development. In oral language pointing becomes increasingly verbally coded by deictic markers (this, that, you);[85] in ASL early pointing becomes differentiated into several different usages: demonstrative pronoun (that), determiner (the), part of the possessive system (my, your), reflexive (self), plural (more than one), and specific reference (this one).[86] Just as crying coexists with later developing forms of oral language, so too does pointing for the deaf. To misinterpret any hand movement that looks to a nonsigner as "just pointing" would be similar to a deaf person's misinterpreting any oral activity as crying or babbling.

In a small study of three hearing and one deaf (of deaf parents) children between 9 months and 2½ years, Volterra analyzed spontaneous gestures used in communication with adults. She discusses two types of gestures: deictic gestures like pointing, showing, and giving; and referential gestures that symbolically represent actions on or functions of an object. Volterra found that all four children used similar gestures of first the deictic and then the referential kind. Referential gestures "often specify what was at an earlier stage referred to only through pointing or other deictic gestures. . . . These signs [sic] pass through the same decontextualization process as words, and become true symbols only at the end of this process."[87] Similar results were obtained by Caselli[88] in a study of six children (8 to 24 months). All the children began to string deictic gestures together or to combine them with a referential sign, but the hearing children also combined a deictic or referential gesture and a word (and presumably would ultimately combine words with words). What differentiated the deaf child from his speaking peers was a developing ability to combine referential signs with each other. One can see in Volterra's preliminary analysis and in Caselli's study the common gestural source of both oral and sign language acquisition as well as the early bifurcation into two different directions determined by the specific medium of communicational input from an adult — either speaking or signing.

Studies of deaf children (of hearing, nonsigning parents) who "spontaneously" develop a "home sign" system seem to argue against the importance of adult guidance, a point of view stressed by Goldin-Meadow and her colleagues[89] in their study of six deaf children. The parents of these children (1 year, 5 months to 4 years, 6½ months) were not skilled signers who could gradually expand the language knowledge of their children. Nevertheless, the parents did interact with their children, directing behavior and using gestures. Comparative analyses of child and parent gestures reveal no difference in basic sign types used by both, even though the children used many different gestures and used their gestural repertoires more productively (e.g., in phrases). Even though they seem to express the same semantic relations as the early one and two word utterances described by Brown and others, whether these home sign systems can substitute for early language is not clear. For example, after a similar start in language acquisition, such children demonstrate language delays and gaps in linguistic knowledge, compared to their hearing and speaking peers; these differences increased with age.[90]

Deaf children of hearing parents have the natural endowment for language. Like hearing children, they are ready to encode their experiences symbolically. It would seem that even parents who do not have complete mastery of the symbolic system these children need can influence that early start. Even nonsigning parents can provide the supportive, pragmatic contexts that encourage early language development. At the critical point, however, when more elaborate semantic relations and more complex syntactic patterns become a factor, the lack of shared symbolic system results in loss and delay of continued language growth.

Waiting until deaf children go to school to redress this language delay is to miss critical years during the optimal period for language development. Excessive drill on language structures, typical of remediation with disabled speakers, leads to rote parroting and "dead speech."[91] As mentioned above, in normal development language structures are acquired as children interact with skilled communicators, creating contexts where language serves a purpose. Lack of knowledge of appropriate contextual constraints brands speakers as outsiders. At Gallaudet College deaf students who were socialized in the hearing world had difficulty, even after learning ASL, in understanding the contexts of appropriate use for signing. Recent signers were unable to capture the subtle variations "of formation, vocabulary and grammatical rules depending on the participants in the conversation, the subject being discussed, the formality or informality of the setting and other social variables."[92] Beyond knowledge of grammatical rules (syntax), to be able to use language appropriately (pragmatics) requires having learned it in meaningful contexts. Jones and Quigley[93] describe two hearing children of deaf parents who developed full parallel bilingual competence in both ASL and English, without interference between the two languages. Both languages were clearly used in specific contexts; both were valued and encouraged because they accomplished communicational ends.

Examining sign language acquisition, one finds parallels to oral language development in content, structures, sequencing, and uses. Following similar stages, early gesturing becomes symbolic, used to express early semantic relations; syntactic structures become increasingly complex. As with mastery of any symbol system, possibilities open up for new categories, for metaphoric extension and change. Signers acquire the ability to use signs appropriately in more and more complex settings.

Signing mothers respond just as speaking mothers do, sometimes imitating their children's immature or incorrect language, other times correcting or expanding it.[94] Signing mothers adjust their language to meet their children's more limited linguistic capacities.[95] Signing children repeat their mother's signs and make mistakes in early "articulation" of signs similar to those made by speaking children. It has even been suggested that signing children using two hands to "duplicate" gestures may be doing motorically what young speakers often do verbally: *tum-tum* for *stomach* or *tummy*, *bye-bye* for *goodbye*, *choo-choo* for *train*. Such reduplication is common in speech by and for young children everywhere. Future studies will delineate more of the details of similarities and differences in the acquisition of oral and sign languages.

Some differences between oral and sign language development have been mentioned in several studies. One is the use of signs by babies as young as 5 months. Another is the purportedly increased vocabulary size in very young signers, compared to their speaking peers. Reports of babies of 5 months signing *milk* would predate oral first words by several months. One 19-month-old child studied by Schlesinger and Meadow had 117 signs, as compared to between 3 and 50 words for a typical hearing-speaking age-mate.[97] Another study of 11 children of deaf parents learning sign as their primary language found evidence of accelerated early language development.[98] Studies of the acquisition of sign language will tell us more about children's language abilities as a function of modality.[99]

One reason that deaf signing children may be more advanced initially in vocabulary is that signing may map more directly onto the gestures that all children are using in preverbal communication. Mothers may be able to interpret gestures as signs and to shape them into signs, as speaking-hearing mothers do with early words. Another factor may be that manual dexterity develops earlier than articulatory motor skills. Piaget and other developmentalists[100] have noted early hand and eye-hand coordination. Additionally, the cognitive underpinnings to language, hypothesized by Piaget as sensorimotor intelligence, develop according to him as a result of the child's active manipulation of objects in the environment. To the degree that early acquired signs are tied to actions on objects or by objects (as some theorists claim) these signs may be more easily learned. However, contrary to some hypotheses,[101] there is no evidence that first signs acquired are necessarily more iconic in nature.[102]

That signs may begin by being more closely tied to gestures does not preclude their functioning ultimately as symbols. Words are not initially symbolic for hearing-speaking children, but only gradually become so. Vygotsky, for example, states that the internal or symbolic relationship between sign and referent develops gradually, building upon an earlier external relationship between word and object in which the word functions as an attribute or a property of the object.[103]

In light of recent theoretical considerations, the importance of a communication system between mother and child in the early years cannot be stressed enough — not just to enable the child to acquire a symbol system (i.e., a language) but to enable full psychosocial development. Schlesinger and Meadow, using an Eriksonian framework, discuss how deaf children master the sequential conflicts that typify developmental changes (e.g., trust versus mistrust, autonomy versus shame and doubt).[104] In all cases deaf children of deaf parents exhibit less conflicted, better adjustments, while deaf children whose hearing parents did not encourage or use manual communication fared worse. The two key factors that make a difference, cited by Schlesinger and Meadow, are greater and quicker acceptance of a deaf child's disability by deaf parents and their concomitant willingness to use manual communication.

Deaf children, especially of hearing parents, can suffer serious disadvantages in early communicational interactions with their mothers. Mothers' expectations of their deaf babies as potential communicators are curtailed; deaf children do not send out cues that the mother can interpret. Typically, hearing parents recognize or suspect deafness in their offspring much later than deaf parents. Deaf babies may vocalize or babble for some months before stopping, leading hearing parents to expect "normal" responses and to be baffled and frustrated by the differences their babies exhibit, even before deafness is diagnosed. Nor can mothers of deaf children tell if their messages are being received. The whole rhythm of communication can be disturbed. Although every mother alters her communication and interaction to fit her perception of her child's limitations due to immaturity, she does so from some sense of what it is like to be an infant. The difficulty parents of a deaf child have in accepting and dealing with their child's additional limitation may arise from a real lack of understanding of a deaf child's experience. The communicational ability of a hearing mother of a deaf child may become strained since she does not "know from the start what it will take [for her son or daughter] to speak the native language"; nor can she "treat the child's efforts from the start as if he [or she] were a native speaker or were soon to be."[105]

It may be for these reasons that authors often describe deaf persons as immature in caring for others, egocentric and lacking in empathy, and impulsive without controlled behavior.[106] A symbol system is necessary to establish true intersubjectivity — shared meanings and shared intention.[107] Emphasis on introducing language early into the world of deaf infants has its roots in two uses of language: cognitive and emotional-social. To enable full cognitive development, some symbolic communication is necessary; but to enable full emotional development, the importance of communication in the earliest period of a child's life is equally critical.[108]

In summary, then, it may be said that the young deaf child has both the capacity for language and the cognitive beginnings on which language competence can be built. The additional determinant is interaction in dialogues with skilled users of language to express all its functions. We now know that sign languages like ASL can serve as that language. Sign languages are not only as structurally complex and complete as oral languages, but they can function as a symbolic, social medium of communicational intent. Used comfortably by mother and child to construct communication contexts, sign languages can establish the social and psychological relationships out of which linguistic, cognitive, and communicational proficiencies naturally emerge. Compared to this natural acquisition, the explicit teaching of language forms devoid of functional contexts and psychosocial relationships is artificial, belabored, and never as successful. Research shows that the best signers are those who sign earliest;[109] proficiency can be linked not only to more years of signing practice, but also to signing at a socially and psychologically optimal period and to the use of signing for all language functions. Therefore, the best response for a deaf child in a hearing world is to be multilingual.

REFERENCES

1. Bruner, J. S. (1983). *Child's talk: Learning to use language.* New York: W. W. Norton and Co.

2. *Ibid.*, 18.
3. Kaye, K., and Charney, R. (1980). How mothers maintain 'dialogue' with two-year-olds. In D. R. Olson (Ed.), *The social foundations of language and thought: Essays in honor of Jerome S. Bruner,* (pp. 211–230). New York: W. W. Norton & Co. p. 227.
4. Eimas, P. D., Siqueland, E. R., Jusczyk, P., and Vigorito, J. (1971). Speech perception in infants. *Science, 171,* 303–306. Spitz, R. A., and Wolf, K. M. (1946). The smiling response. A contribution to the ontogenesis of social relations. *Genetic Psychology Monographs, 34,* 57–125. Fantz, R. L. (1967) Visual perception and experience in early infancy. In H. Stevenson, E. Hess, and H. Rheingold (Eds.), *Early behavior: Comparative and developmental approaches.* New York: Wiley & Sons. An excellent review of early infant studies can be found in Stone, L. J., Smith, H. T., and Murphy, L. B. (Eds.) (1973, 1978). *The Competent Infant Series,* Basic Books.
5. Beginning in 1957 with *Syntactic Structures.* The Hague: Mouton. More fully elaborated in 1965, *Aspects of the Theory of Syntax.* Cambridge, MA: MIT Press.
6. Bloomfield, L. (1933). *Language.* New York: Holt, Rinehart and Winston. p. 39.
7. Lenneberg, E. H. (1962). Understanding language without ability to speak: A case report. *J. Abnormal Soc. Psychol, 65,* 419–425.
8. Hockett, C. F. (1963). The problem of universals in language. In J. H. Greenberg (Ed.), *Universals of Language* (2nd ed., pp. 1–29). Cambridge, MA: MIT Press. pp. 8–13.
9. Neville, H. J., and Bellugi, U. (1978). Patterns of cerebral specialization in congenitally deaf adults: A preliminary report. In P. Siple (Ed.), *Understanding language through sign language research* (pp. 293–257). Poizner, H., and Buttison, R. (1980). Cerebral asymmetry for sign language: Clinical and experimental evidence. In H. Lane and F. Grosjean (Eds.), *Recent perspectives on American Sign Language* (pp. 79–101). Hillsdale, NJ: Lawrence Erlbaum.
10. Siple, P. (1982). Signed language and linguistic theory. In L. Menn and L. Obler (Eds.), *Exceptional language and linguistics* (pp. 313–318). New York: Academic Press. Stuttert-Kennedy, M. (1980). Language by hand and by eye. *Cognition, 8,* 93–108. Grosjean, F. (1981). Sign and word recognition: A first comparison. *Sign Language Studies, 32,* 195–220.
11. Conrad, R. (1979). *The deaf schoolchild: Language and cognitive function.* London: Harper & Row. Brooks, P. H. (1979). Some speculations concerning deafness and learning to read. In L. S. Liben (Ed.), *Deaf children: Developmental perspectives* (pp. 87–101). New York: Academic Press. Nickerson, R. S. (1979). On the role of vision in language acquisition by deaf children. In L. S. Liben (Ed.), *Op. cit.* (pp. 115–134). On the processing of the man-

ual alphabet in finger-spelling, see Hoemann, H. W. (1978). Categorical coding of sign and English in short-term memory. In P. Siple (Ed.), *Op. cit.* (pp. 289–304).

12. Klima, E. S., and Bellugi, U. (1975). Perception and production in a visually based language. In D. Aaronson and R. W. Rieber (Eds.), *Developmental psycholinguistics and communication disorders* (pp. 225–235). New York: New York Academy of Sciences. p. 230.

13. Mindel, E. D., and Vernon, M. (1971). *They grow in silence*. Silver Spring, MD: National Association of the Deaf. p. 53.

14. Klima, E. S., and Bellugi, U. (1975). *Op. cit.* p. 233. Klima, E. S., and Bellugi, U. (1979). *The signs of language*. Cambridge, MA: Harvard University Press. pp. 317–372.

15. Schlesinger, H. S., and Meadow, K. P. (1972). *Sound and sign*. Berkeley: University of California Press. Hoffmeister, R., and Wilbur, R. (1980). The acquisition of sign language. In H. Lane and F. Grosjean (Eds.), *Op. cit.* pp. 61–78.

16. Klima, E. S., and Bellugi, U. (1979). *Op. cit.* Stokoe, W. C. (1978). *Sign language structure*. Silver Spring, MD: Linstok Press. Wilbur, R. (1976). The linguistics of manual language and manual systems. In L. Lloyd (Ed.), *Communication assessment and intervention strategies* (pp. 423–500). Baltimore: University Park Press. Wilbur, R. (1979). *American Sign Language and sign systems*. Baltimore: University Park Press.

17. Wilbur, R. (1979). *Op. cit.*

18. Fischer, S. (1978). Sign language and creoles. In P. Siple (Ed.), *Op. cit.* (pp. 309–331). Woodward, J. (1978). Historical bases of American Sign Language. In P. Siple (Ed.), *Op. cit.* (pp. 333–348). See also *Sign Language Studies*, 1972 to the present, for a series of articles on pidgin ASL and on ASL as pidgin and creole.

19. For a provocative analysis of the relationship between creolization and child language, with implications for ASL, see Bickerton, D. (1981). *Roots of language*. Ann Arbor: Karoma Publishers. Bickerton (1982) focuses on "the [linguistic] achievements of children, who could not have been taught by mother, since mother herself did not know the language her children would acquire." (Learning without experience the creole way. In L. Menn and L. Obler [Eds.], *Op. cit.* [pp. 15–29]. p. 16.)

20. On changes in sign language over generations, see Newport, E. L. (1981). Constraints on structure: Evidence from American Sign Language and language learning. In W. A. Collins (Ed.), *Aspects of the development of competence.* (Minnesota Symposia on Child Psychology, Vol. 14, pp. 93–124). Hillsdale, NJ: Lawrence Erlbaum.

21. Hamalian, L. (1965). Communication by gesture in the Middle East. *ETC. A Review of General Semantics, 22*, 43–49.

22. Bates, E., Camaioni, L., and Volterra, V. (1975). The acquisition of performatives prior to speech. *Merrill-Palmer Quarterly of Behavior and Development, 21,* 205–226. Kaye, K. (1982). *The mental and social life of babies.* Chicago: University of Chicago Press. Bates, E. (1976). *Language and context: The acquisition of pragmatics.* New York: Academic Press. Bruner, J. S. (1975a). From communication to language. *Cognition, 3*(3), 255–287. Bruner, J. S. (1975b). The ontogenesis of speech acts. *Journal of Child Language, 2,* 1–19. Lock, A. (1978). (Ed.). *Action, gesture and symbol.* New York: Academic Press.

23. Clark, E. V. (1978). From gesture to word: On the natural history of deixis in language acquisition. In J. Bruner and A. Garton (Eds.), *Human growth and development* (pp. 85–120). Oxford: Oxford University Press. Wales, R. (1979). Deixis. In P. Fletcher and M. Garman (Eds.), *Language acquisition* (pp. 241–260). Cambridge: Cambridge University Press.

24. Barten, S. S. (1979). Development of gesture. In N. R. Smith and M. B. Franklin (Eds.), *Symbolic functioning in children* (pp. 139–151). Hillsdale, NJ: Lawrence Erlbaum.

25. Bloomfield, L. (1933). *Op. cit.,* p. 39.

26. Rommetveit, R. (1974). *On message structure: A framework for the study of language and communication.* New York: Wiley & Sons.

27. deVilliers, J. G., and deVilliers, P. A. (1978). *Language acquisition.* Cambridge, MA: Harvard University Press. p. 238.

28. Sigel, I. E., and Cocking, R. R. (1977). *Cognitive development from childhood to adolescence: A constructionist perspective.* New York: Holt, Rinehart, and Winston.

29. Tervoort, B. (1961). Esoteric symbolism in the communicative behavior of young children. *American Annals of the Deaf, 106,* 436–480.

30. de Saussure, F. (1959). *Course in general linguistics.* New York: Philosophical Library. p. 66.

31. deVilliers, J. G., and deVilliers, P. A. (1978). *Op. cit.,* p. 239. Bellugi, U., and Stuttert-Kennedy, M. (Eds.). (1980). *Signed and spoken language: Biological constraints on linguistic form.* Weinheim: Verlag Chemie. See also note 10.

32. Klima, E. S., and Bellugi, U. (1979). *Op. cit.*

33. Ibid.; Bellugi, U., Klima, E. S., and Siple, P. (1975). Remembering in signs. *Cognition, 3,* 93–125. Grosjean, F. (1980). Psycholinguistic: Psycholinguistics of sign language. In H. Lane and F. Grosjean (Eds.), *Op. cit.* (pp. 33–59). Newkirk, D., Klima, E. S., Pedersen, C., and Bellugi, U. (1979). Linguistic evidence from slips of the hand. In V. Fromkin (Ed.), *Slips of the tongue and hand.* Proceedings of the 12th International Congress of Linguistics, Vienna.

34. Markowicz, H. (1980). Myths about American Sign Language. In H. Lane and F. Grosjean (Eds.), *Op. cit.* (pp. 1–6). Klima, E. S. and Bellugi, U. (1979). *Op. cit.*, pp. 7–83.

35. Bruner, J. S. (1973). The growth of representational processes in childhood; The course of cognitive growth. In J. M. Anglin (Ed.), *Beyond the information given: Studies in the psychology of knowing* (pp. 313–351). New York: W. W. Norton & Co.

36. Moores, D. F. (1974). Nonvocal systems of verbal behavior. In R. L. Schiefelbusch and L. L. Lloyd (Eds.), *Language perspectives — Acquisition, retardation and intervention* (pp. 402–403, 407). Baltimore: University Park Press. Mindel, E. D., and Vernon, M. (1971). *Op. cit.*, pp. 75–76.

37. Ibid.

38. Vygotsky, L. S. (1962). *Thought and language.* Cambridge, MA: MIT Press. pp. 61, 75.

39. Ibid., 69.

40. Ibid., 38.

41. Vygotsky, L. S. (1978). *Mind in society: The development of higher psychological processes.* (M. Cole, V. John-Steiner, S. Scribner, and E. Souberman, Eds.). Cambridge, MA: Harvard University Press.

42. Moores, D. F. (1974). *Op. cit.*

43. Meadow, K. P. (1980). *Deafness and child development.* Berkeley: University of California Press.

44. Padden, C., and Markowicz, H. (1982). Learing to be deaf: Conflicts between hearing and deaf cultures. *The Quarterly Newsletter of the Laboratory of Comparative Human Cognition, 4* (4), 67–72.

45. Lou, H. C. (1982). *Developmental neurology.* New York: Raven Press.

46. Lenneberg, E. H. (1967). *Biological foundations of language.* New York: Wiley & Sons. Lenneberg, E. H., Rebelsky, C. F., and Nichols, I. A. (1965). The vocalizations of infants born to deaf and to hearing parents. *Human Development, 8,* 23–37. For an alternate view, see Gilbert, J. H. V. (1982). Babbling and the deaf child: A commentary on Lenneberg et al. (1965) and Lenneberg (1967). *Journal of Child Language, 9,* 511–515.

47. Oller, D. K. (1985). Infant vocalizations: Traditional beliefs and current evidence. In S. Harel and N. J. Anastasiow (Eds.), *The at-risk infant: Psycho/socio/medical aspects* (pp. 323–331). Baltimore: Paul H. Brookes Publishing Co. Oller, D. K., Eilers, R. E., Bull, D. H., and Carney, A. E. (1985). Prespeech vocalizations of a deaf infant: A comparison with normal metaphonological development. *Journal of Speech & Hearing Research, 28,* 47–63. Oller, D. K., and Bull, D. H. (1984). *Vocalizations of deaf infants.* Presented as a poster session at the International Conference on Infant Studies, New York.

48. Even under conditions of limited input (e.g., with amplification), deaf infants share many features of younger hearing infants' vocalizations. Larger samples of deaf infants in future studies will explore how generalizable and how predictive of later speech these findings are.

49. Feldman, H., Goldin-Meadow, S., and Gleitman, L. (1978). Beyond Herodotus: The creation of language by linguistically deprived deaf children. In A. Lock (Ed.), *Op. cit.* (pp. 351–414). Goldin-Meadow, S. and Feldman, H. (1977). The development of language-like communication without a language model. *Science, 197*, 401–403. Goldin-Meadow, S. (1979) Structure in a manual communication system developed without a conventional language model: Language without a helping hand. In H. Whitaker and H. Whitaker (Eds.) *Studies in neurolinguistics* (Vol. 4, pp. 125–209) New York: Academic Press.

50. Goldin-Meadow, S. (1982). The resilience of recursion: A study of a communication system developed without a conventional language model. In E. Wanner and L. R. Gleitman (Eds.), *Language acquisition: The state of the art* (pp. 52–77). Cambridge: Cambridge University Press.

51. Morehead, D. M., and Morehead, A. (1974). From signal to sign: A Piagetian view of thought and language during the first two years. In R. L. Schiefelbusch and L. L. Lloyd (Eds.), *Op. cit.* (pp. 153–190).

52. Furth, H. G. (1966). *Thinking without language.* New York: Free Press. Furth, H. G. (1969). *Piaget and knowledge.* Englewood Cliffs, NJ: Prentice-Hall. Furth, H. G. and Youniss, J. (1976). Formal operations and language: A comparison of deaf and hearing adolescents. In D. M. Morehead and A. E. Morehead (Eds.), *Normal and deficient child language* (pp. 387–410). Baltimore: University Park Press.

53. For example, Sinclair-de-Zwart, H. (1969). Developmental psycholinguistics. In D. Elkind and J. Flavell (Eds.), *Studies in Cognitive Development* (pp. 315–336). New York: Oxford University Press.

54. Brown, R. (1973). *A first language.* Cambridge, MA: Harvard University Press.

55. Schlesinger, H. S. and Meadow, K. P. (1972). *Op. cit.* Hoffmeister, R., and Wilbur, R. (1980). *Op. cit.*

56. Vygotsky, L. S. (1962). *Op. cit.* Zaporozhets, A. V., and Elkonin, D. B. (Eds.). (1971). *The psychology of preschool children.* Cambridge, MA: MIT Press.

57. Moores, D. F. (1974). *Op. cit.* pp. 406–409. Moores, D. F. (1978). Current research and theory with the deaf: Educational implications. in L. S. Liben (Ed.), *Op. cit.* (pp. 173–193). pp. 182–184.

58. Zaporozhets, A. V., and Elkonin, D. B. (1971). *Op. cit.*

59. Litowitz, B. E., and Litowitz, N. S. (1983). Development of verbal

self-expression. In A. Goldberg (Ed.), *The future of psychoanalysis* (pp. 397–427). New York: International Universities Press.

60. Mahler, M. S., Pine, F., and Bergman, A. (1975). *The psychological birth of the human infant.* New York: Basic Books.

61. Spitz, R. A. (1963). The evolution of dialogue. In M. Shur (Ed.), *Drives, affects, behavior* (Vol. 2, pp. 170–190). New York: International Universities Press. Spitz, R. A. (1963). Life and the dialogue. In H. S. Gaskill (Ed.), *Counterpoint* (pp. 154–176). New York: International Universities Press.

62. Halliday, M. A. K. (1975). *Learning how to mean: Explorations in the development of language.* London: Edward Arnold. Halliday, M. A. K. (1973). *Explorations in the functions of language.* London: Edward Arnold.

63. Freedman, D. A. (1981). Speech, language and the vocal-auditory connection. *Psychoanalytic Study of the child, 36,* 105–127. p. 121.

64. Meadow, K. P., Greenberg, M. T., and Erting, C. (1983). Attachment behavior of deaf children with deaf parents. *Journal of the American Academy of Child Psychiatry, 22* (1), 23–28.

65. Galenson, E., Miller, R., Kaplan, E., and Rothstein, A. (1979). Assessment of development in the deaf child. *Journal of the American Academy of Child Psychiatry, 18,* 128–142.

66. Greenberg, M. T., and Marvin, R. S. (1979). Patterns of attachment in profoundly deaf preschool children. *Merrill-Palmer Quarterly, 25,* 265–279.

67. For example, Uzgiris, I. C. (Ed.) (1979). *Social interaction and communication during infancy.* Washington, DC: Jossey-Bass. Bullowa, M. (Ed.) (1979). *Before speech: The beginnings of interpersonal communication.* Cambridge University Press.

68. Condon, W. S. (1979). Neonatal entrainment and enculturation. In Bullowa, M. (Ed.), *Op. cit.* (pp. 131–148).

69. Stern, D. (1977). *The first relationship: Infant and mother.* London: Fontana/Open Books. Bruner, J. S. (1975a, 1975b, 1983). *Op. cit.*

70. Bates, E., Benigni, L., Bretherton, I., Camaioni, L., and Volterra, V. (1977). From gesture to first word: On cognitive and social prerequisites. In M. Lewis & L. A. Rosenblum (Eds.), *Interaction, conversation and the development of language.* New York: Wiley and Sons.

71. Moerk, E. (1977). *Pragmatic and semantic aspects of early language development.* Baltimore: University Park Press. p. 63.

72. Bruner, J. S. (1974). *Op. cit.,* p. 283.

73. Halliday, M. A. K. (1973, 1975). *Op. cit.*

74. Halliday, M. A. K. (1973). *Op. cit.,* p. 24.

75. Ibid., 27.

76. Ibid., 20.

77. Bruner, J. S. (1983), *Op. cit.* Kaye, K. (1982). *Op. cit.*

78. Kaye, K. (1982). *Op. cit.*, pp. 127, 122, 131.
79. Snow, C. E., deBlauw, A., and Van Roosmalen, G. (1979). Talking and playing with babies: The role of ideologies of child-rearing. In M. Bullowa (Ed.), *Op. cit.* (pp. 269–288). p. 287.
80. Bruner, J. S. (1983). *Op. cit.* Bruner, J. S. (1982). The formats of language acquisition. *American Journal of Semiotics, 1* (3), 1–16.
81. Gleitman, L. R. and Wanner, E. (1982). Language acquisition: The state of the art. In E. Wanner and L. R. Gleitman (Eds.), *Op. cit.* (pp. 3–48). p. 41.
82. Barnes, S., Gutfreund, M., Satterly, D., and Wells, G. (1983). Characteristics of adult speech which predit children's language development. *Journal of Child Language, 10,* (1), 65–84. p. 83.
83. Ibid. 77.
84. For example, Bates, E., Camaioni, L., and Volterra, V. (1975). *Op. cit.* Dore, J. (1974). A pragmatic description of early language development. *Journal of Psycholinguistic Research, 3,* 343–50.
85. Clark, E. (1978). *Op. cit.* Wales, R. (1979). *Op. cit.*
86. Hoffmeister, R., and Wilbur, R. (1980). *Op. cit.* pp. 71–73.
87. Volterra, V. (1981). Gestures, signs and words at two years: When does communication become language? *Sign Language Studies, 33,* 351–361. pp. 353–354.
88. Caselli, M. C. (1983). Communication to language: Deaf children's and hearing children's development compared. *Sign Language Studies, 39,* 113–144.
89. See Note 49.
90. Mohay, H. (1982). A preliminary description of the communication systems evolved by two deaf children in the absence of a sign language model. *Sign Language Studies, 34,* 73–90.
91. Vygotsky, L. S. (1978). *Op. cit.* p. 105.
92. Padden, C. and Markowicz, H. (1982). *Op. cit.* p. 70.
93. Jones, M. L., and Quigley, S. P. (1979). The acquisition of question formation in spoken English and American Sign Language by two hearing children of deaf parents. *Journal of Speech and Hearing Disorders, 44,* 196–208.
94. Compare, Snow, C. E., and Ferguson, C. A. (Eds.). (1977). *Talking to children: Language input and acquisition.* Cambridge: Cambridge University Press with Schlesinger, H. S. and Meadow, K. P. (1972). *Op. cit.*
95. Maestas y Moores, J. (1980). Early linguistic environment: Interactions of deaf parents with their infants. *Sign Language Studies, 26,* 1–13. Kantor, R. (1982). Communicative interaction: Mother modification and child acquisition of American Sign Language. *Sign Language Studies, 36,* 233–282.
96. Barten, S. S. (1979). *Op. cit.* p. 148.
97. Schlesinger, H. S., and Meadow, K. P. (1972). *Op. cit.* p. 56.
98. Bonvillian, J. D., Orlansky, M. D., and Novack, L. L. (1983). Devel-

opmental milestones: Sign language acquisition and motor development. *Child Development, 54,* 1435–1445. However, Caselli's warning should be heeded: "Ascertaining and analyzing the communicative usage of deictic and referential gestures by hearing children has shown the need to compare not just the words of hearing children with the signs of deaf children but in fact, and as a first step, the gestures (especially referential) and words of hearing children with signs of deaf children. Otherwise no valid assessments of similarities and differences in acquisition process can be made. . . . It is not that deaf children begin to communicate earlier, but that both deaf and hearing children use gestural expression earlier in their communication with adults." Caselli, M. C. (1983). *Op. cit.* pp. 141–142.

99. Newport, E. L. (1982). Task specificity in language learning? Evidence from speech perception and American Sign Language. In E. Wanner and L. R. Gleitman, *Op. cit.* (pp. 450–486).

100. Piaget, J. (1963) [1952, IUP]). *The origins of intelligence in children.* New York: W. W. Norton & Co. White, B. L. (1969). The initial coordination of sensorimotor schemas in human infants — Piaget's ideas and the role of experience. In D. Elkind and J. H. Flavell (Eds.), *Studies in cognitive development* (pp. 237–256). New York: Oxford University Press. Bruner, J. S. (1969). Eye, hand and mind. In D. Elkind and J. H. Flavell (Eds.), *Studies in cognitive development* (pp. 223–235). New York: Oxford University Press.

101. Brown, R. (1979). Why are signed languages easier to learn than spoken languages? In E. Carney (Ed.), *Proceedings of the National Symposium on Sign Language Research and Teaching.* Silver Spring, MD: National Association of the Deaf.

102. Bonvillian, J. D., Orlansky, M. D., and Novack, L. L. (1983). *Op. cit.*

103. Vygotsky, L. S. (1962). *Op. cit.* p. 28.

104. Schlesinger, H. S. and Meadow, K. P. (1972). *Op. cit.* Erikson, E. H. (1968). *Identity, youth and crisis.* New York: W. W. Norton & Co.

105. Bruner, J. S. (1978). Learning how to do things with words. In J. Bruner and A. Garton (Eds.), *Op. cit.* (pp. 62–84). p. 83.

106. Schlesinger, H. S., and Meadow, K. P. (1972). *Op. cit.* p. 2. Meadow, K. P. (1980). *Op. cit.* Harris, R. I. (1978). Impulse control in deaf children: Research and clinical issues. In L. S. Liben (Ed.), *Op. cit.* (pp. 137–156).

107. Kaye, K. (1982). *Op. cit.*

108. Edgecumbe, R. M. (1981). Towards a developmental line for the acquisition of language. *The Psychoanalytic Study of the Child, 36,* 71–103. Freedman, N. and Grand, S. (1977) (Eds.). *Communicative structures and psychic structures.* New York: Plenum. Galenson, E., Kaplan, E. H., and Sherkow, S. (1983). The mother-

child relationship and preverbal communication in the deaf child. In J. D. Call, E. Galenson, and R. L. Tyson (Eds.), *Frontiers of infant psychiatry* (pp. 136–149). New York: Basic Books.

109. Mayberry, R., Fischer, S., and Hatfield, N. (1983). Sentence repetition in American Sign Language. In J. G. Kyle and B. Woll (Eds.), *Language and sign*. London: Croom Helm.

CHAPTER 8

After the Revolution: Educational Practice and the Deaf Child's Communication Skills

Rachel Mayberry
Rhonda Wodlinger-Cohen

T he past 15 years have witnessed a radical rethinking about how and where deaf children are educated. Dramatic change has taken place in the way teachers communicate to their deaf students. Equally great change has occurred in where deaf children are educated in relation to their families and normally hearing peers. When the first edition of this book was published, 85 percent of severely and profoundly deaf children in the United States were enrolled in schools that used a strictly oral method of communication in the classroom (that is, speech communication with absolutely *no* kind of accompanying manual communication permitted — sign, fingerspelling, or cues).[1] Now, 15 years later, 95 percent of special programs for deaf children have reported using some kind of simultaneous speech and manual communication in the classroom.[2] Fifteen years ago, 48 percent of all school-age deaf students attended classes away from home in residential schools, whereas in 1984, 74 percent attended day classes while living at home. Similarly, in 1984 15 percent of deaf students attended regular classes with normally hearing students on a full-time basis, and an additional 21 percent on a part-time basis; 15 years ago the practice was sufficiently rare that no figures are available.[3,4] Changes of this magnitude in so little time are revolutionary.

What are the outcomes of the revolution? To some extent it might be too early to tell. Many diverse elements of the educational system must accommodate the change, such as teacher preparation and training, parent education, and administrative policy. In addition, the educational system may still be reacting to the revolution. Observations we make now may be inaccurate later after the educational system has made even more accommodation. Nevertheless, enough time has passed to observe groups of deaf children who first began their education after key elements of the revolution were in place. The time has come to ask some initial questions as to how the communication system used with deaf children affects their communication skill development.

In this chapter we will address in detail several specific and related questions about educational practice and the deaf child's communication skills. First, does the age at which the deaf child first learns sign language affect the eventual proficiency with which he or she can understand and use it later in adulthood? Second, are hearing teachers capable of speaking and signing at the same time when they communicate to deaf students? Third, how does the amount of sign language available in the home environment affect the deaf child's development of communication skills? Fourth, can the deaf child learn the artificial language of signed English as well as the natural language of American Sign Language? Last, how does the deaf child's sign language ability relate to reading ability? Before discussing the answers we have found during our investigations of the deaf community and classrooms for deaf children, we will briefly describe the various elements of the revolution, including the controversy over communication methods used in deaf children's classrooms and recent legislative and judicial decisions affecting their education.

EDUCATIONAL PRACTICE

What Motivates Educational Practice?

We are often asked why the education of deaf children generates such heated controversy among professionals. There is unfortunately no easy answer to this question. Sharp clashes of opinion may be endemic to deaf education simply because its various educational practices are grounded in assumptions that are basically contradictory. To complicate matters, many motivations underlying the education of deaf children are value judgments and therefore not resolvable through empirical means of inquiry and proof. Perhaps this is one reason why the methodological controversy in deaf education has continued unabated for the past 2 centuries.

Educational practice is influenced by a myriad of sources, including the way in which teachers and administrators are trained to teach, their response to their own educational experience, what they believe to be the goal and purpose of education, and their experience with the product of their teaching efforts. For teachers of deaf children, this means that their educational methods are influenced and guided by their professional training in deaf education, personal experience with individuals who are deaf, and — perhaps most important — what they believe to be the best educational outcome for the deaf student.[1] Thus the educator who believes that the most successful deaf person is one who can speak will teach very differently from the educator who believes that the ability to speak is unimportant to the deaf person's success.

Equally germane is the fact that educator's beliefs about the value of speech are based, in turn, on complex theoretical and philosophical assumptions about the nature and structure of language. All educational methods used in classrooms for deaf children arise from deep-seated beliefs as to exactly what language is, how it is structured, and how children come to know it, or more accurately, how hearing children develop the ability to produce and understand language. Educators agree that severe and profound deafness isolates infants, toddlers, and children from the spoken language that surrounds them so that their learning of it is grossly impeded. Educators disagree, however, as to what it is that deaf children need to learn. Is it speech that deaf children lack, or language? Is speech the same thing as language, or is it a vehicle for language? If speech is a linguistic vehicle, separable from language itself, then what is the best supplement to or substitute for speech? These questions are complex, and educators of deaf children are not the only ones who grapple with them; scholars, too, are deeply divided over these questions.

Communication Mode and
Educational Practice

The educational literature commonly debates the pros and cons of various teaching methods from the standpoint of sensory mode, the question being whether one set of sensory stimuli can adequately serve as a substitute for another in the child's language development. Here the question is usually whether vision can substitute for audition. In the following discussion of educational methods, we will follow suit and focus first on teaching methods that rely on audition and then on those that rely on vision. We will not exhaustively describe and discuss every educational method that has been and is currently being used to teach deaf children language. Rather, we will selectively describe only some teaching methods in order to illustrate the way in which differing beliefs about the nature of language can lead to the exclusive use of different sensory modes for classroom communication.

Auditory Communication

Auditory methods of teaching deaf children language, more commonly known as "oral" methods, are based on a number of assumptions. The list includes, among others, beliefs that (1) the ability to speak affords the deaf person the greatest number of educational and employment options; (2) speech is the same thing as language; (3) good speech skills are necessary in order to develop good reading skills; (4) speech proficiency is best achieved early in life; and (5) the deaf child's development of speech will be impeded if he or she also communicates via nonspeech means — nonspeech communication will lessen the incentive to practice the more difficult skill (namely speech) and thus limits how much the child will practice speaking. Although these basic assumptions underlie all methods of auditory-oral education, they are variously instantiated in educational practice.

UNISENSORY COMMUNICATION. One method of oral education, known as the *acoupedic* or *unisensory* approach, is based on the assumptions that (1) children learn language by listening to it; (2) nonauditory means of language learning will fail to bring about complete language skill; and (3) auditory perceptual skill can be developed in any child whose hearing is impaired, provided the training is begun at a sufficiently early age with the aid of amplification and the child's parents are willing to carry out the auditory training at home.[5] Because auditory perceptual ability is being developed, this method discourages the child from supplementing or substituting other sensory perceptions for listening, such as the use of vision in speechreading. Teaching efforts are therefore directed solely at auditory stimulation and perception in the absence of other sensory cues.

MULTISENSORY SPEECH PRODUCTION. Another method of oral education is based on the assumption that children learn language through speech production. The multisensory method assumes that the *oral motor patterns* of speech are the building blocks of the structure of language and are learnable by children who cannot hear provided that they are given sufficient and explicit teaching and extensive practice; speech learning must begin early in life with the aid of amplification. The method also assumes that the deaf child's parents are willing to evoke and guide the child's speech production at home. Unconscious and exact speech production is the teaching goal of this approach developed by Ling,[6] but, unlike the unisensory approach, the speech goal is accomplished through listening in conjunction with other sensory cues as deemed necessary by the teacher to bring about precise speech, such as cues using vision and tactition.

These two approaches, one aurally based and the other orally based, illustrate clearly the direct effect that different beliefs about the nature of language and about how children learn it have on the way deaf children are taught. Thus the substance of any two given methods can be radically different from one another, despite identical goals (in the above two cases, intelligible speech). Generally the implementation of oral education is not as explicit and narrow as the above two examples imply, but rather is a mix of several teaching methods, all designed to foster the deaf child's development of auditory reception and speech production skills without recourse to any visual means of communication other than speechreading and written language.

Visual Communication

For the child who is deaf, auditory perception is impaired but vision usually is not. Consequently, a common practice of deaf educators is to capitalize on this fact in teaching language to deaf children. Such methods presume that the ability to know and understand language is more important to the deaf child than is the ability to speak intelligibly. These methods assume that complete focus on and attention to speech — production or reception — can impede the deaf child's language development because the time and attention devoted to speech (a skill the child may never acquire) replace the time and attention available for language (something no child should be without). Visual approaches to communication assume that the major handicap of deafness is a reduced or absent ability to *receive* or *perceive* language and that the handicap is reduced if language is made receivable and perceivable. A fundamental belief underlying visual approaches is that the sensorimotor form of language is less crucial to the language learning process than is the linguistic structure and content of the language input. These approaches typically stress language *input* — regardless of its sensorimotor form — assuming that input plays a causal role in a child's language development and that language production will be a naturally occurring consequence of language input as long as the form of the input is perceivable.

Several teaching methods have been designed to capitalize on the deaf child's intact visual system by replacing or simultaneously supplementing the auditory portion of speech with visual hand gestures. There are many different ways this might be accomplished, but the most common are cued speech, fingerspelling, and simultaneous communication, the last method encompassing sign language.

SPEECHREADING. Speechreading first comes to mind as a kind of visual language, but by itself, speechreading is not a successful means for teaching language. Individuals unfamiliar with deafness often mistakenly believe that the movements made by the mouth during speaking are a complete, visual counterpart to speech (just as print represents speech) so that mouth movements can provide the deaf child with a viable means of learning spoken language. However, decades of teaching deaf children have shown that mouth movements alone give only a very incomplete picture of speech acoustics. Successful speechreading is due more to good guesses as to which words and phrases are being spoken than to visual recognition of speech sounds. Thus, people who lost their hearing after having learned language are generally better speechreaders than those born deaf or who became deaf before learning the language. Research has shown that hearing adolescents who have never had a single speechreading lesson are better speechreaders than congenitally deaf adolescents who have had continuous speechreading instruction since early childhood.[7] Speechreading is a skill that rides piggyback on prior language knowledge. The visual portion of speech by itself provides young deaf children with insufficient exposure to language to enable them to learn it spontaneously as young hearing children do by listening.

CUED SPEECH. Cued speech was created to fill the gaps left by the visual mouth movements of speech.[8,9] Lip and mouth movements are supplemented with manual cues designed to help the speechreader distinguish among speech sounds that look identical on the lips (i.e., homophones). The cues consist of eight different handshapes made in four different positions around the mouth and are shown in Figure 8–1. One handshape in one position signals an entire set of speech sounds. The speech sounds within each of the handshape sets all look different on the lips. Thus it is impossible to identify specific speech sounds on the basis of the cues alone or on the basis of the mouth configuration alone. The mouth configuration together with the cue constitutes the visual representation of the speech sound. This approach assumes that the acoustic signal of speech can be fully and best represented for the deaf child by two types of visual information, mouth configuration and manual cues. The approach further assumes that a visual model of this sort can adequately serve as a substitute for acoustic language input, so that the deaf child can learn language in the same fashion as does the child who can hear, but by watching rather than by listening.

FINGERSPELLING. Cued speech was devised only recently as a means of making spoken language available to deaf children; fingerspelling has been available as a supplement to, or replacement for, spoken language for as long as 400 years.[10] Fingerspelling serves as a visual substitute for speech at an entirely different level of representation than any of the previously discussed communication methods and modes. Rather than representing speech, fingerspelling represents writing. The American (including Canadian) fingerspelling system consists of 26 hand-

CUED SPEECH
American English

CHART I
Cues for Vowel Sounds

	Side	*Throat*	*Chin*	*Mouth*
open	ah (father) (got)	a (that)	aw (dog)	
flattened-relaxed	u (but)	i (is)	e (get)	ee (see)
rounded	oe (home)	oo (book)	ue (blue)	ur (her)

CHART II
Diphthongs

ie (my)	ou (cow)	ae (pay)	oi (boy)

CHART III
Cues for Consonant Sounds

t	h	d	ng	l	k	b	g
m	s	p	y	sh	v	n	j
f	r	zh	ch	w	dh	wh	th
				z			

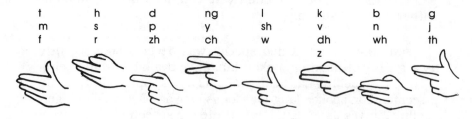

Figure 8–1. *The handshapes and positions of Cued Speech. (From R. O. Cornett, Cued Speech Office, Gallaudet College, Washington, D.C. Adapted by permission.)*

156

shapes, each representing one letter of the alphabet, as shown in Figure 8–2. To produce a word, the fingerspeller gestures a handshape for each letter of the word just as he or she would write it. Used as a means of teaching deaf children language, fingerspelling is commonly referred to as the *Rochester method* because it was first used and promoted for this purpose in the United States at the Rochester School for the Deaf in New York.[11] In its execution, the Rochester method resembles cued speech because the speaker talks while simultaneously gesturing with one hand held close to the mouth. In fingerspelling, the speaker gestures the letters of the words rather than the sounds. The assumptions underlying the Rochester method are (1) knowing language is more important than speaking, and language can be represented visually as well as acoustically; (2) by fingerspelling everything said to the child, the child has the opportunity to learn language by perceiving a full and complete model of spoken language; (3) the content of the language model is more important than the form of the representation, and it makes no difference that written letters are gestured rather than some portion of the acoustic signal of speech.

SIMULTANEOUS COMMUNICATION. *Sign and Speech.* All visual means of classroom communication discussed up to this point involve the simultaneous generation of visual-gestured and acoustic-spoken input. The gestured portion of the communication methods vary in terms of the level of spoken language which is represented — speech sounds, sound features, or written letters. In the communication method known as *simultaneous communication,* speech is also produced simultaneously with manual gestures, but here the gestures represent the words and grammatical units of spoken language. This is accomplished by adopting and modifying the sign language that has evolved among deaf people themselves. In the United States this sign language is known as American Sign Language (ASL).

Sign language has always been used extensively by deaf people for communication, despite the fact that educators actively prohibited it from schools and classrooms for a very long time (a policy that has changed only within the past decade). Sign language is often mistakenly thought of as having been invented by teachers of deaf children to represent spoken language, but in fact recent research has shown that deaf children are the originators of sign language. Deaf children show a strong propensity to develop their own gestural systems even when

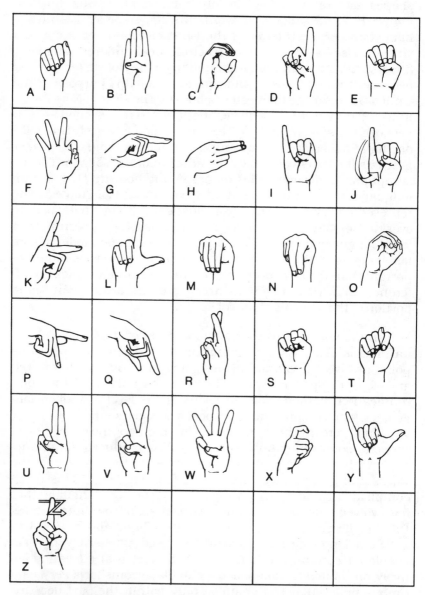

Figure 8–2. *The handshapes of American Fingerspelling. (From International Hand Alphabet Charts (2nd ed., p. 77) by S. Carmel 1982, published by the author. Copyright 1982 by S. Carmel. Reprinted by permission.)*

158

there is no sign language available to them in the environment.[12] This fact demonstrates that the drive to communicate is as strong in the deaf child as it is in the hearing child. It is highly probable that ASL has evolved over the centuries from deaf children's gestural systems. Only later did some teachers of deaf children stumble on the idea of adopting and modifying the colloquial sign language of deaf people as a means of teaching spoken language.[13] ASL has a linguistic structure that is quite different from English (see, for example, Klima and Bellugi, 1979; Wilbur, 1979)[14,15] so that extensive modifications are necessary in order to make it comparable to English.

In simultaneous communication the deaf child is both signed and spoken to at the same time with the assumption that the child will develop either or both modes of communication depending upon his or her predilections and abilities. The signed portion of the communication consists of signs taken from ASL and designed to represent English words, as well as numerous invented and adopted signs designed to represent English vocabulary and bound morphemes (grammatical markers such as past tense, plural, possessive, etc.). These invented and adopted signs are frequently amalgams of ASL signs and fingerspelling; a new sign is generated by changing the sign's handshape to correspond to the initial letter of an English word as it would be written (see, for example, Gustason, Pfetzing, and Zawolkow, 1972).[16]

The assumptions underlying this method are quite similar to those of the other visually based methods. First, the method assumes that it is possible to adequately represent spoken language in vision. However, in simultaneous communication the gestures represent the words and morphemes of spoken language. Second, the method assumes that the deaf child can learn language in the same fashion as does the child who can hear, albeit through a combination gestured and spoken language, as long as the deaf child is provided with a complete and frequently occurring visual language model.

In sum, we see that one major disagreement among educators of deaf children is whether speech should be the focus of educational efforts, or whether language in general should be the goal. Moreover, even when educators agree on the goal, important differences in method still remain. Over the 1½ decades, more and more schools have abandoned strict adherence to oral methods and tried, for the first time, signing in the context of simultaneous communication. The change in educational practice was the consequence of several factors: First was a greater societal acceptance of ethnic groups and minority languages. Second was a general dissatisfaction on the part of teachers, parents, and deaf adults with the academic achievement of deaf students. Third was increased knowledge and understanding of sign language.

Another force that has been instrumental in bringing about the recent revolutionary change in educational practice has been the intervention of the law into educational matters. Before we consider the impact this change in educational practice has had on the deaf child's communication skills, we will describe the recent legislation and judicial decisions that have altered how deaf children are taught.

LEGISLATIVE DECISIONS AND EDUCATIONAL PRACTICE

In the 1960s Americans began to acknowledge that the rights of minority groups were not being recognized; attempts were made to remedy the situation through federal legislation mandating that the civil rights of minorities not be violated. Society's growing awareness that equal treatment was each individual's birthright, regardless of race, religion, sex, age, or national origin, soon broadened to encompass individuals whose handicaps prohibit them from participating in mainstream society. Two pieces of federal legislation in particular were important forces in the recent revolution in educational practice for deaf children. First was the Rehabilitation Act, and second was the Education of All Handicapped Children Act.

The Rehabilitation Act

In 1973 Congress passed the Rehabilitation Act, commonly known as Section 504, which states,

> No otherwise qualified individual in the United States . . . shall, solely by reason of his [or her] handicap, be excluded from participation in, be denied the benefit of, or be subject to discrimination under program of activity receiving federal financial assistance. *United States Congress, Section 504 of the Rehabilitation Act of 1973, Public Law 93-112.*[17]

Scope

For individuals who are deaf the law serves to prohibit job discrimination and provide equal access to any public service provided by any office or agency receiving federal funds. The prohibition against job discrimination is identical in its inception and enaction to the civil rights protection extended to members of minority groups; the equal access provision of the law, however, requires unique accommodation for the deaf person. For deaf people who use sign language, this means that educational, medical, and social agencies receiving federal funds must provide sign language interpreters so that deaf employees, consumers, and clients can participate in and receive their services to the same extent as people who are not deaf.

The law has especially served to open many previously closed doors to deaf people who use sign language, such as hospitals and clinics, police stations and courts, and colleges and universities. The law has also spawned a corps of professionally trained sign language interpreters, the Registry of Interpreters for the Deaf. The law requires equal access but leaves the method of access up to each individual agency; consequently there is great variability in accessibility of public services to deaf people. Some agencies have instituted fast-acting systems to obtain sign language interpreters when the need arises — others behave as if the law did not exist or as if they have never encountered sign language or a deaf person who uses it. Full participation in mainstream society, despite federal legislation, often requires an enormous amount of persistence and diligence on the part of the deaf person. However, the mere existence of the law gives the deaf person some concrete means of demanding and fighting for equal treatment in society.

Recent Judicial Modification

In 1984 the Supreme Court narrowed the interpretation of the federal prohibition against sex, race, and age discrimination (Title IX of the Education Amendments of 1972). Unless new legislation is passed, the narrower interpretation will apply to Section 504 as well.[18] The Court decided (*Grove City College v. Bell*)[19] that federal antidiscrimination law need only apply to specific programs within institutions that receive federal funds. Generalized to Section 504, this means that a college must provide a sign language interpreter to a deaf student only in those departments that directly receive federal monies. A college would be required to provide an interpreter for psychology courses if the psychology department received federal grants, but not for literature courses if the English department received no direct federal support. According to Strauss,[18] in 1985 the U.S. Department of Education dropped more than 60 investigations of alleged institutional discrimination against handicapped individuals as as consequence of the recent Supreme Court ruling. This narrow and specific interpretation of Section 504 wreaks havoc with the spirit and concept of equal access to publicly supported services by handicapped citizens; new legislation is sorely needed that will unify and generalize antidiscrimination law throughout entire institutions and agencies.

Education of All Handicapped Children Act

More germane to the education of deaf children in the United States was the passage in 1975 of the Education of All Handicapped Children Act, more commonly known as Public Law 94-142, which states,

It is the purpose of this act to assure that all handicapped children have available to them . . . a free appropriate public education which emphasizes special education and related services designed to meet their unique needs, to assure that the rights of handicapped children and their parents or guardians are protected, to assist states and localities to provide for the education of all handicapped children, and to assess and assure the effectiveness of efforts to educate handicapped children (*United States Congress, Education of All Handicapped Children Act of 1975, Public Law 94-142).*[17]

Scope.

The federal government mandated that all public educational facilities receiving federal funds make their services available to handicapped children between the ages of 3 and 21 years. The law gives general guidelines as to how public school systems are to provide educational service to handicapped children, including the rights of handicapped children and their families to participate in the educational planning process by having their wishes, suggestions, and objections fairly and objectively considered and treated.

Specifically, the law states that the education of each handicapped child must be designed and implemented to meet that particular child's needs; the child's family must be allowed to participate with the school in meeting these needs. This is accomplished in several ways.

First, each handicapped child's educational needs and the way the school will meet these needs is outlined in an individualized educational program (IEP).[17] The IEP is reviewed yearly by both the child's teachers and his or her parents or guardians. The IEP specifies the child's current level of functioning and expected improvement. It also outlines short-term instructional goals for the following year.

Second, the law states that the IEP for each handicapped child must be based on nondiscriminatory evaluation and testing conducted every 3 years, or more frequently if needed, by a multidisciplinary team. The testing team must include at least one teacher or specialist knowledgeable about the handicap. Further, the testing must be conducted in the child's native language or communication mode and be geared to assess the child's specific educational needs in terms of strengths or weaknesses.

Third, the law further states that if the parents or guardians object to the IEP or the evaluation, they can request a due process hearing. A due process hearing is an informal meeting between the child's parents or guardians and school officials conducted by a neutral third party known as a hearing officer.[20] The hearing officer, following specific procedures set by each state, receives and reviews the information regarding the child and his or her current placement and educational needs as presented by both the school and the child's parents or guardians. The child's family has a right to have a lawyer present, to call witnesses who are experts in educating handicapped children, to ask questions, and to request an independent educational evaluation. After considering all the presented evidence and information, the hearing officer determines the appropriate placement for the child. The decision is final unless it is appealed to the state department of education or the courts.

Judicial Interpretation

In 1982 the Supreme Court heard its first case relevant to the Education for All Handicapped Children Act. The dispute involved the education of a profoundly deaf child (*Hendrick Hud-*

son Central School District v. Rowley).[21] In this case the parents requested that their child be provided with a sign language interpreter so that she could better understand her teachers, but the school disagreed, saying that the child was doing well without an interpreter. The Court decided in favor of the school, citing evidence that the child was making adequate progress in a regular classroom for normally hearing students even without an interpreter. The Court's decision narrowed the interpretation of the law to mean that public school systems must provide a "free and appropriate education" specific to each handicapped child, but that they need not educate each handicapped child to the maximum of his or her potential.[22] At the same time, however, the Court upheld the basic tenets of the law, namely that each handicapped child has a right to (1) individualized instruction, (2) support services (at public expense) necessary to benefit from education, (3) parental or guardian involvement in the development of IEPs, and (4) due process and judicial review in the case of disputes.[23]

A natural fear of educators, families, and deaf adults was that either the law or the Court's recent decision would result in judicial decisions by lower courts or actions taken by educational agencies in favor of specific educational methodologies or kinds of educational settings across the board without regard or sensitivity to the varying needs of each deaf child. For example, the courts and educational agencies might decide that all deaf children should be educated solely in neighborhood public schools or that no deaf student should have an interpreter. However, after analyzing a number of judicial cases involving Public Law 94-142, DuBow and Geer[22] have found that this has not happened. The courts have focused on the "individualized education" requirement of the law. As a consequence, an equal number of cases have been decided in favor of the parents as in favor of the schools. Some cases have been resolved in the placement of deaf children in residential schools and some in regular public schools. Likewise, in terms of methodological questions, such as whether spoken or signed language or cued speech should be used with the deaf child, the courts have arrived at a variety of decisions, each reached as a result of the evidence presented in support of what would best benefit the child given his or her current level of functioning and need for improvement. Sometimes these communication and methodological decisions have upheld the families' wishes and sometimes not.

DuBow and Geer[22] observe that the key factor in the recent judicial decisions involving deaf children has been the weight of evidence presented in support of the recommended placement by specialists who knew the child well. They also observe that the courts have not decided in favor of philosophical preferences of schools or parents that are presented without documented evidence in terms of the deaf child's strengths, weaknesses, and needs. The fear that mixing the law and education might produce one-sided or superficial educational services for the deaf child has not been borne out.

Federal law has had significant impact on the practice of educating deaf children and on their potential freedom to participate in society at large after they grow up. Only 15 years ago, nearly half of all deaf children attended school while they lived apart from their families. Today, nearly 74 percent are able to live with their families and attend school at the same time. Estimates vary, but approximately 36 percent of deaf children participate with normally hearing children in academic activities at least half of the time.[4,24] Much of this change can be attributed to the mixing of law and education. Whether the overall effect has been a positive or negative force on the academic achievement of deaf children remains to be seen.

Next we examine the product of past and recent educational practice by observing and analyzing some of the communication skills of deaf adults and children, in addition to those of hearing teachers.

THE DEAF CHILD'S COMMUNICATION ENVIRONMENT AND SKILLS

What kind of difference does educational methodology make in the deaf child's development of communication? We intuitively see that both the environment and education play an important role because the worst possible circumstances, such as an environment that contains little or no communication interaction coupled with little or no education, produce two devastating consequences for the child born severely or profoundly deaf: Social and cognitive isolation. But aside from the worst possible case, to what extent is specific educational practice responsible for specific communication outcomes? For example, if a profoundly deaf child becomes an intelligible speaker, is this the product of the way in which he or she was taught? If the deaf child does not achieve this skill despite specific and intense instruction, is the method at fault, or does the child lack some unidentified special speech capacity? Similarly, if a deaf student becomes a proficient reader and writer, is this notable success the unique product of personal endowment, independent of the educational circumstances in which fate placed the child, or can the child's school and teachers take full credit? Obviously these questions are neither unique to deaf children and their education nor readily answerable. Indeed, these questions, in a more general form, have plagued philosophers and educators for centuries.

The Office of Demographic Studies at Gallaudet College, after years of collecting and analyzing the academic achievement scores of deaf students nationwide, has found two factors in particular to be especially good predictors of a deaf child's academic success. The first is the degree to which the child can hear. The second is the income level, or socioeconomic status, of the child's family.[25] These factors are indelible from an educational standpoint: Schools cannot alter these facts, but rather must work with them. Given these boundaries, then, what do we know about the relationship between educational practice and development of communication skills? We will approach this question primarily from the standpoint of sign language.

Research Questions

During the past 5 years we have been examining and analyzing the relationship between the amount and kind of communication present in the deaf child's environment and the proficiency with which the child can understand sign language. Of course, sign language is only one part of a constellation of communication skills used and taught in classrooms for deaf children, but it is important to study its development for several reasons. Sign language is the communication mode about which we know the least, but at the same time is the communication mode most commonly used by deaf adults. Moreover, sign language is currently a key element in the educational practice of simultaneous communication.

We began our research with the assumption that a relationship exists between the development of the deaf child's communication skill (in this case sign language) and the extent to which particular kind of communication is available in the deaf child's home and school environment. We have found that this relationship is not a simple one, and, in addition, that several common beliefs about sign language learning are false.

Age Limitations on Learning Sign Language

In describing some of the assumptions underlying various modes and methods of teaching language to deaf children, we have noted that several "oral" or "nonmanual" approaches to educational practice are motivated by the belief that spoken language is best learned early, that is, early in childhood as opposed to after childhood. The hypothesis is not new, but has been a common tenet of language research for the past 20 years.[26] In the field of deaf education, the hypothesis provided a major impetus for the widespread development of early identification and intervention programs for deaf infants and children and their families.

Usually when we think of a childhood advantage for language learning, we think of the advantage in terms of spoken languages such as English, French, and Spanish. Commonly the children in immigrant families learn the language of the new country without a trace of an accent, but the parents engage in an interminable struggle with the language, often never mastering it. If we think of sign language as being gestural or pantomimic — not language — then anyone should be able to master it at any age. However, if we regard sign language as being linguistic, another kind of language, then we might expect the same maturational constraints to apply to the learning of sign language as apply to the learning of spoken language. Ironically, the past educational practice of deaf educators in the United States has inadvertently provided a natural experiment by which we can determine whether the childhood advantage for language learning applies to sign language as well as to spoken language.

Past Educational Practice

Recall that 85 percent of schools for the deaf in the United States practiced oral education exclusively until as recently as 15 years ago. This means that no kind of sign language or gesture was used by either the teachers or the students in the classroom, and that parents were actively discouraged from learning or using sign language at home. Thus, a majority of deaf children had the opportunity to learn sign language only if and when they were placed in an environment where they could see it — most commonly at a residential school. In dormitories, deaf children were exposed to and learned sign language from those few deaf children who came from deaf families, or sometimes from deaf house parents. Until about 15 years ago, educators actively

and uniformly kept deaf children from seeing sign language during early childhood in the hope that this practice would promote
and facilitate learning of speech. Only after educators decided
that a student could not learn to speak was the deaf student
transferred to a residential school and thus permitted to see sign
language. This decision was frequently made after the deaf student was no longer a child. The result of this long-standing educational practice is that the older population of deaf signers in
the United States varies widely with respect to how old they were
when they first learned to sign. Does this variation in learning
circumstance affect the ability of deaf signers to understand and
use sign language?

*The Consequences of Age of Acquisition on Memory for
Sign Language*

We are conducting several studies designed to examine the
relationship between the age at which deaf signers first learned
to sign and the proficiency with which they can understand sign
language in later adulthood. In one study, we asked deaf college
students to give verbatim recall of simple ASL sentences.[27,28] We
grouped the signers in terms of the age at which they first
learned to sign, ranging from birth to 15 years. Most of the signers first learned to sign in the situation described earlier, sign
language immersion in the dormitory. The results showed that
the younger the signer when he or she first began to sign, the
more accurate the performance.

Possibly, though, sign language takes an especially long
time to learn; the signers might have shown more equal sign language ability if they all had had the same amount of experience
with sign language, independent of the age of initial exposure.
To test the hypothesis, we replicated the study with a group of
older, more experienced, deaf signers who had not attended
college.[29,30,31] In this second study, the signers again varied in
terms of the age at which they first learned to sign (most learning sign language in the dormitory immersion situation), but in
this case all of the signers had used sign language as a primary
means of communication for a comparable and extensive
amount of time, 35 years or more. We asked the signers to recall
another, more complex, set of ASL sentences. Again the results
showed a significant correlation between the age at which the
signer first learned to sign and performance accuracy on the
task: The younger the signer when he or she began to learn to

sign, the more accurately he or she reproduced the meaning of ASL sentences.

The effect of age of acquisition on signers' ability to remember only the meaning or both the form and the meaning of ASL sentences is remarkably consistent across the two studies, as is shown in Figure 8–3. Despite the fact that the signers in the first study had far less total experience (6 to 20 years) than did those in the second study (35 to 50 years), the effect of age of acquisition on memory for sign language is nearly identical. Moreover, the effect is nearly identical despite the fact that the proficiency measures differ in the two studies: in the first study the measure was accuracy of verbatim recall, and in the second the measure was accuracy of meaning recalled. Newport has similarly found an effect of age of acquisition on the proficiency with which deaf signers are able to produce various grammatical structures in ASL. These studies suggest that the learning of sign language is guided by the same sort of developmental guideposts as is the learning of spoken language.

For reasons we do not yet understand, young children are more efficient language learners (in sign language or spoken language) than older children, adolescents, or adults. Although educators of deaf children have tried to take this fact into account

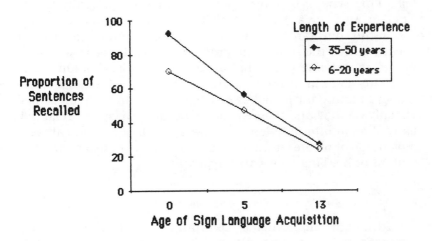

Figure 8–3. *The short-term memory accuracy for ASL sentences by deaf signers as a function of the age at which they first learned to sign and the length of time they have signed.*

in their past efforts to teach spoken language, they have not always done so in the case of sign language. Sign language, perhaps because it is visual and gestured, has been considered by educators to be a "safety net" for the deaf child; that is, educators have considered sign language to be a communication system for which the deaf student has unbounded learning potential, regardless of age. If a deaf student fails to learn to speak and speechread, educators have assumed that the child can learn sign language at any subsequent time. There is, however, no evidence to support this reasoning. On the contrary, the result of past educational practice demonstrates that language must be learned early in life to be learned well, no matter whether it is spoken and listened to or gestured and watched.

Is Simultaneous Communication Possible?

Deaf children were kept from seeing sign language in the past so that teaching efforts early in the child's life could be devoted to spoken language. In addition, educators recognized that ASL was not English. As we briefly described earlier, ASL has a different vocabulary and grammatical structure than does English. One important factor in the recent proliferation of signing in classrooms for deaf children was the advent of a kind of signing that, although based on ASL, was designed to represent English. This type of signing is known as either Manually Coded English (MCE) or, as we shall call it here, *signed English.*

In the simultaneous method of communication, the teacher speaks and at the same time produces a sign for each word and bound morpheme (or grammatical marker). The rationale behind this communication method is that it provides an accessible and redundant model of English — one that is represented visually on the hands (signs) and on the mouth (speechreading), as well as auditorially (speech). As a result the child can take advantage of whatever mode or combination of modes that best suit his or her language learning proclivities.

Criticisms of Simultaneous Communication

Although simultaneous communication has been widely implemented in classrooms for deaf children, the extent to which it succeeds at providing an adequate model for the language learning child has been seriously questioned for a number of different reasons. Most objections revolve around the fact that signed English is artificial. Rather than having evolved like a natural language through human usage and learning, signed English was invented at meetings by educators. We know that all children are well equipped to learn natural languages, but we do not know whether — or how — they learn artificial ones. The distinction is potentially very important.

Research has shown that sign language, specifically ASL, has evolved to fit the hands and eyes well[33] in the very same sense that spoken language has evolved so that speakers are not required to produce sounds that the mouth cannot make or the ear cannot perceive. The invented signs used in simultaneous communication are often ones that would never be found in a natural sign language because they require the signer to make awkward hand and arm movements, or movements that are difficult or impossible to detect visually. A related criticism is that signed English requires the signer to produce too many signs in too little time. Bellugi and Fischer[34] observed that signing an isolated ASL sign takes about twice as long as saying an isolated English word. Simple calculation suggests that simultaneous production of sign and speech is temporally impossible. Something must be changed, and it must be either that speech production is significantly slowed or that a significant number of signs are omitted. Another criticism of simultaneous communication relates to the fact that, because ASL is visual and three-dimensional, it marks word and grammatical categories with changes in sign shape, movement or location; this spatial nature is destroyed in simultaneous communication when each sign must be paired with a spoken word or morpheme. Together these criticisms suggest that simultaneous communication does not provide an adequate model for language learning because it gives only a very poor picture to the eye and distorted speech to the ear. Perhaps we should question whether simultaneous communication is even producible by teachers before we ask whether it enables deaf children to learn language.

Teachers' Production of Simultaneous Communication

Marmor and Petitto[35] observed the simultaneous communication of two teachers, each of whom had approximately 3 years' experience communicating in this fashion. The deaf students they taught ranged in age from 11 to 13 years. Analyzing the teachers' speech and sign production separately, Marmor and Petitto observed that their spoken utterances were primarily grammatical (93 percent and 89 percent), but that they failed to accompany each word they spoke with a sign. These findings have been used in support of the claim that simultaneous communication, especially the signed portion, is impossible to produce and therefore does not provide the deaf child with a grammatical language model. More recently, however, Wodlinger-Cohen[36] has found that the way in which teachers produce simultaneous communication is much more complicated and systematic than these earlier findings suggest.

Wodlinger-Cohen observed and described the simultaneous communication of normally hearing teachers of three different-aged classes of deaf children (5, 10, and 14 years) in day schools. The teachers in her study were not novices, but had 5 to 10 years of practice using simultaneous communication. Analyzing together the speech and signed portions of the teachers' utterances, she found that the teachers spoke grammatical English more than 99 percent of the time. When she further analyzed the teachers' signed representation of their speech, she found a regular pattern of variation. As the age of the deaf students increased, the teachers decreased the proportion of spoken morphemes they accompanied with signs. In other words, the teacher of the five-year-olds simultaneously accompanied nearly each spoken morpheme with one signed morpheme, whereas the teacher of the 10-year-olds produced fewer accompanying signs, and the teacher of the 14-year-olds produced the least number of accompanying signs. Additional analyses showed that the teachers did not omit signs haphazardly, but rather omitted signs as a function of morpheme type. As Figure 8–4 shows, the teachers were most likely to represent open-class morphemes (vocabulary or content words, such as *boy, car,* or *drive*) simultaneously in speech and sign, less likely to represent closed-class morphemes (grammatical markers that stand alone, such as *the* or *his*) with an accompanying sign, and least likely to produce signs for bound morphemes along with speech (grammatical markers on the ends of words, such as *–s,* or *–ed*).

Note that the fewer the closed- and bound-class morphemes the children produced in either speech or sign, the more likely their teacher was to produce these morphemes (see Figure 8–4). This finding suggests that the less sophisticated the deaf child's English, the more complete the English model the teacher provides on her hands to accompany her speech. Conversely, the more sophisticated the deaf child's English, the less complete the English model the teacher provides on her hands. This relationship, in fact, suggests that the teachers observed by Marmor

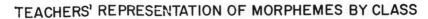

TEACHERS' REPRESENTATION OF MORPHEMES BY CLASS

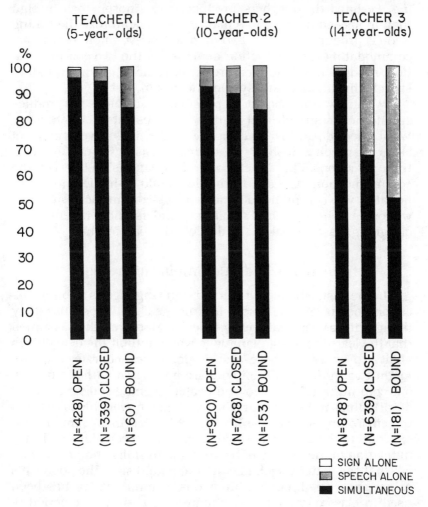

Figure 8–4. *Teachers' representation of morpheme types as a function of communication mode.*

and Petitto omitted signs because of the age and linguistic sophistication of the deaf students they taught rather than because simultaneous communication is impossible to produce.

Contrary to theoretical speculation, Wodlinger-Cohen's findings show that it is possible for teachers of deaf children to produce communication simultaneously in speech and sign and, moreover, that the way they do so is highly sensitive to the age and linguistic sophistication of the deaf students they are teaching. Perhaps the teachers produce fewer morphemes in sign than in speech in order to equalize and synchronize the timing of their production in the two modes. However, note that in accommodating the production demands of the two communication modes, the teachers are nevertheless grammatical in speech and linguistically systematic in sign.

We know now that it is possible for teachers to produce simultaneous speech and sign as they instruct deaf children. What effect does this have on the deaf child's development of skills in speech and sign? We approach this next question from three directions. First we examine the relationship between the communication available to the deaf child at home and his or her ability to comprehend simultaneous communication. Then we contrast the deaf child's ability to understand different kinds of signing. Last we look at the deaf child's reading skills.

The Deaf Child's Communication Skills

In the past, educators reserved sign language as a communication means of last resort for the deaf child because they thought it was especially easy to learn. Moreover, they assumed that the learning of sign language would inhibit the deaf child's ability to speak. If these assumptions are accurate, then we might expect deaf children who are instructed with simultaneous communication to show equivalent signing skills regardless of variations in the amount of sign language available to them in the environment (because it is "easy" to learn). We might also expect that the quality of the deaf child's speech skills will vary in relation to the quality of his or her sign skills and, in particular, that the better the child can understand sign, the poorer his or her speech will be. Simultaneous communication has been used in classrooms for deaf children for a sufficient period of time now to enable us to test these hypotheses.

General Study

We have studied the ability of deaf students to understand stories presented three ways: Simultaneous communication (speech and signed English), ASL, and print. We were especially interested in determining whether a relationship exists between the amount and kind of sign language available to the deaf child in the environment and the development of reading and signing abilities.[37] All the deaf students tested and observed have been enrolled from the beginning of their schooling in educational programs that employed and encouraged the use of simultaneous communication both in the classroom and at home.

Students Living in Hearing Households

Of the children studied ranging in age from 7 to 15 years, 26 lived at home with normally hearing families. As might be expected, the hearing parents and guardians varied in terms of whether or not they accompanied their speech with signs when they communicated to their deaf children. In the group we studied, 23 percent (6 students) reported that both of their hearing parents or guardians usually produced signs simultaneously with speech when in direct communication with them at home. More commonly, the student reported that only his or her mother produced signs with speech and that no one else at home used any sign; this was the situation for 54 percent of the group (14 students). Some students reported that no one in the family used signs when they spoke; this was the case for 23 percent of the group (6 students). All the students from hearing households attended the same schools and had the same teachers, so that the primary difference among their communication environments was the amount of sign they saw at home.

Students Living in Deaf Households

We also observed and tested another group of deaf students, but these all lived in deaf households where their deaf parents (and in some cases deaf siblings) communicated with them primarily in sign language and rarely in signed English. These students attended the same classes and were taught by the same teachers as the group from normally hearing households, and were matched to the first group on the basis of age, sex, and IQ.

Environment and Communication Skill

For the deaf students living in hearing households, we first analyzed the relationship between the amount of sign in their homes and their ability to understand simultaneous communication. We began by sorting the students into three different home communication categories: Sign input from two adults, sign input from one adult, and no sign input. In general, we found that the deaf students who received sign input from two adults at home were more likely to develop good skills in comprehending simultaneous communication (in comparison to their aged-matched peers) than students who received sign input from only one adult or none at all. Similarly, students who received no adult sign input at home were unlikely to develop above-average comprehension of simultaneous communication in relation to their age-matched peers.

We found no relationship between the amount of residual hearing the deaf students possessed and the likelihood that their hearing parents or guardians signed to them. We expected that the hearing parents would be more likely to sign to their child the less the child was capable of hearing, but this was not the case among these students, whose hearing losses were severe and profound. In the same vein, the students who had intelligible speech were as likely to be signed to by their parents and guardians as were those who did not speak intelligibly or had no speech at all. These last two findings suggest that a deaf child's ability to hear or speak are not the factors that motivate the child's hearing parents or guardians to sign when speaking to him or her.

In terms of speech ability, 30 percent of the deaf students from hearing households had speech that was intelligible. Interestingly, the students with intelligible speech also showed skill in comprehending simultaneous communication. Thus the belief that understanding sign impedes the development of speech production appears to be false.

What about the students' ability to understand the signed English used in simultaneous communication as contrasted to ASL? Because the parents and guardians of the students from hearing households have primarily communicated with their deaf children in either speech alone or speech accompanied by signs, we would expect these students to understand signed English, but not ASL, with which they have had significantly less experience. At the same time, however, critics have charged that signed English, not being a natural language, may not be learnable. If this is the case, we would expect the students from both the hearing and the deaf households to show little understanding of signed English and simultaneous speech. Last, we would expect that the students from the deaf households to be able to understand ASL because their parents have used it to communicate with them at home. Additionally, there is a possibility that their ability in ASL might interfere with their ability to understand signed English because ASL has a wholly different linguistic structure from signed English.

We found no support for any of these hypotheses when we looked at the students' abilities to understand stories given in simultaneous speech and signed English as contrasted to ASL. First, we found that the students from hearing households can and do learn to understand simultaneous speech and signed English. These students' ability to understand the stories given in signed English and simultaneous speech increases as they get older, as Figure 8–5 shows. These same students also show some ability to understand the stories given in ASL, and this ability also increases with age (see Figure 8–5). Thus, all the groups of students from hearing households can understand signed English, and they can also understand — to a lesser degree — ASL.

The students from deaf households, like their peers from hearing households, show an ability to understand signed English and simultaneous speech, an ability that increases as they grow older, as Figure 8–5 shows. The youngest group of students from deaf households, 7 to 9 years of age, show nearly equivalent understanding of signed English and ASL (see Figure 8–5), whereas the oldest students from deaf households, 13 to 15 years, show a greater understanding of ASL than of signed English. Note, however, that although the oldest students from deaf households show greater understanding of ASL than signed English, their ability to understand signed English is equal to or greater than that of their age-matched peers from hearing households. This suggests that the additional amount of sign language input that the students from deaf households receive, even though it has a different linguistic structure than English, facilitates rather than impedes their comprehension of signed English and simultaneous speech.

An important feature of the students' developing ability to understand stories given in sign alone (ASL) and simultaneous speech and sign (signed English) is that the advantages of a home environment rich in sign language are not yet apparent in the performance of the youngest students, who are 7 to 9 years old, but rather show up when the students are a few years older. This may reflect the magnitude of the language learning task that confronts the deaf child. The deaf students here are learning to understand English in the forms of speech, sign, and print, in addition to another language, ASL.

These results suggest several important points for our discussion of educational practice. First is that the signed English of simultaneous communication, contrary to theoretical criticism, does appear to be learnable by deaf children whose teachers use this mode of communication with them. The students

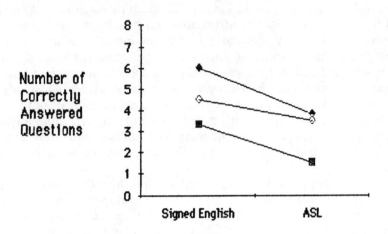

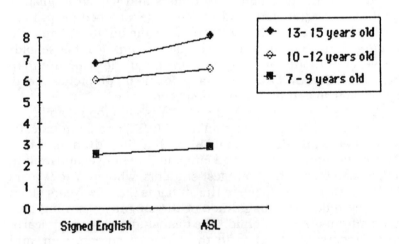

Figure 8–5. *The comprehension of stories given in signed English (and simultaneous speech) and ASL by deaf students, grouped by age and parental hearing status.*

from hearing and deaf households understand this kind of communication even though it was designed by committee rather than evolved through community usage. Second, the use of a non-English-based sign language in the home, ASL, does not appear to interfere with the deaf students' ability to learn and understand the signed English of simultaneous communication. Last, these findings suggest that the amount of conversational interactions that the deaf child engages in throughout his or her development contributes as much to the growth of comprehension ability as does the specific kind of grammatical structure through which the conversations take place.

Signing Skills and Reading Development

One communication skill of the deaf child to have escaped the scrutiny of researchers and educators until quite recently has been the ability to read. People unfamiliar with deafness are surprised to learn that the child born severely and profoundly deaf is unlikely to read well no matter what language is taught.[38,39] The Office of Demographic Studies reports that the average reading level of deaf students when they leave school at the age of 19 hovers at the fourth grade level,[40] and worldwide data show similar reading levels for deaf students learning other languages in other countries.[38]

Why is reading such a difficult task for the deaf child? There are at least two hypotheses to consider. The first is that reading an unknown language is difficult, so that not knowing English well may be one reason why deaf children often fail to learn to read well. Unlike young hearing children, who have great facility with spoken language when they begin to learn to read, deaf children have comparatively little knowledge of the spoken language encoded in print. A second explanation is that print symbolizes speech sounds; the deaf child may have special difficulty learning to decipher and remember printed words. An early task confronting the young hearing reader is learning to associate the letters printed on the page with the sounds they represent. Having learned to sound out printed words, the child can then decipher words already known in speech but not yet seen in print. We do not know how deaf children circumvent these problems in learning to read, but we know that some do. If these problems were insurmountable, there would be no successful readers among deaf children, and this is not the case.

We may wonder how communication through sign affects the deaf child's reading development. If familiarity with speech is the only avenue to successful reading, then we would expect the reading abilities of deaf students to vary in direct relation to their speech abilities. If, however, knowing the linguistic structure of the language represented in print is of prime importance to the development of reading skill, regardless of whether the language knowledge is in spoken or signed form, then we would expect the reading abilities of deaf students to parallel their abilities in signed English, but not in ASL.

We have examined the reading skills of the students from hearing and deaf households with two separate measures: The Reading Comprehension subtest of the Stanford Achievement Test for Use with Hearing Impaired Students[41] and a written short story comparable to those we gave the students in signed English and ASL.[37] Overall we found that the reading abilities of the deaf students increased with age, as Table 8–1 shows. Five students, or 19 percent, of this group read at a grade level commensurate with their age. An additional two students, or 7 percent, read only one grade level below expectation for their age. This is superior reading achievement in comparison to the deaf school-age population nationwide. This shows that it is possible for the deaf student to read well, but how does this happen, and why does it happen for so few students? If we understood the ingredients that make for successful reading skill in the deaf student, then we might be able to develop teaching techniques that are more appropriate for the special problems the deaf child encounters in learning to read.

We examined the interrelationships among the hearing, speech, and reading abilities of the deaf students from hearing households because a majority of deaf children (more than 90 percent) come from these types of homes. Among these students, we found no relationship between amount of residual

Table 8–1
Deaf Students' Reading Skill Given in Grade Levels

Age	7 to 9 Years		10 to 12 Years		13 to 15 Years	
	Mean	Range	Mean	Range	Mean	Range
Hearing households	2.2	1.0–2.9	4.4	2.1–6.9	4.9	2.7–8.8
Deaf households	2.4	2.1–3.2	5.5	3.3–7.1	6.2	3.5–8.2

hearing and reading ability, and no relationship between speech ability and reading ability. Students whose speech was judged unintelligible were as likely as those whose speech was judged intelligible to show good reading skills in relation to their age-matched peers. Similarly, the few students whose only speech skill was vocalization were as likely as those with intelligible speech to read well.

Among all the students, from both hearing and deaf households, we found a strong relationship between ability to understand signing in the context of *either* signed English or ASL and ability to read. Thus, the greater the student's comprehension ability in either signed English or ASL, the greater his or her reading comprehension. We previously found that students who received no sign input at home were unlikely to develop above-average sign comprehension skills in comparison to their age-matched peers. It follows that these same students were also unlikely to develop excellent reading skills. Recall that the students from deaf households showed a greater average ability to understand both the signed English of simultaneous communication and ASL at older ages than did age-matched students from hearing households. It is therefore not surprising they also showed a greater average reading ability than did their age-matched peers from hearing households even though the sign language they saw and used at home was not English.

Clearly, much more work is needed to understand how deaf children who sign learn how to read. These preliminary results show, however, that for students who are severely and profoundly deaf and are being educated with simultaneous communication, hearing and speech skills are not the major factors that contribute to the development of their ability to read. Understanding language well, either as signed English and simultaneous speech or ASL, appears to play an important role in the deaf child's reading development.

SUMMARY

We have seen that prior to the past decade deaf children were all taught spoken language without the aid of sign language in the beginning of their schooling, sometimes living at home, but most often separated from their families. We have also seen that most deaf children currently are taught spoken language with the continuous aid of sign in a wide variety of settings close to and away from home in classes with both deaf and hearing peers. The change in communication method was a response by the educational system to the demands of teachers, parents, and deaf adults. The change in educational setting was a response by the educational system to society's attempt to bring about equal opportunity through legislative mandate.

Finally, we have seen that several well-entrenched beliefs about the learning of sign language and its relationship to the deaf child's development of other communication skills are false. First, sign language, like spoken language, is best learned early in life; the early years of a deaf child's life that are lost to language learning cannot be recouped by the learning of sign language. Second, teachers can produce simultaneous speech and sign, and in doing so they speak in grammatical English and sign in a linguistically systematic fashion. Third, deaf children exposed to signed English and simultaneous speech learn to understand it. How well they learn to do so depends upon the number of people they can sign and talk to. Learning how to read, in turn, can be based on knowing sign, both the English-like sign of simultaneous communication and the non-English-like sign of ASL. The learning of ASL in no way inhibits the ability to understand signed English and simultaneous speech or the reading of English. Last, deaf children who sign can learn to read well. Their ability to do so is not dependent on their ability to speak and hear, but on their ability to understand sign and speech together or sign alone. Although these new pieces of information are only fragmentary in nature, they point out the educational directions that hold the greatest promise in teaching and preparing the deaf child for the arduous task of living a self-sufficient, self-fulfilling, and productive life in the midst of a society full of both good intention and gross misunderstanding.

ACKNOWLEDGMENTS

The research reported here was supported in part by grants from the U.S. Public Health Service (National Institutes of Health, NS204142 and NS17613) and the Canadian Department of Health and Welfare (6605-1855-43) in addition to funds provided by the Medical Faculty of McGill University. Preparation of this chapter was supported by the University of Chicago through funds provided by the Spencer Foundation. We thank the schools, teachers, and especially deaf children and adults who allowed us to intrude on their precious time while we collected the observations and data reported here. We also thank Drucilla Ronchen for help testing subjects, and Susan Goldin-Meadow and Carl Vonderau for helpful editorial comments.

REFERENCES

1. Silverman, R. (1971). The education of deaf children. In L. Travis (Ed.), *Handbook of speech pathology and audiology* (pp. 399–430). New York: Appleton-Century-Crofts.
2. Nober, L. (1985). *Instructional services to hearing-impaired students in the United States: 1984 update.* Paper presented to the International Congress on Education of the Deaf, Manchester, Great Britain, July.
3. *American Annals of the Deaf: Directory of Services.* (1971). *116,* 214.
4. *American Annals of the Deaf: Directory of Services.* (1984). *129,* 188–189.
5. Pollack, D. (1984). An acoupedic program. In D. Ling (Ed.), *Early intervention for hearing-impaired children: Oral options* (pp. 181–254). San Diego: College-Hill Press.
6. Ling, D. (1976). *Speech and the hearing-impaired child: Theory and practice.* Washington, DC: The Alexander Graham Bell Association for the Deaf.
7. Conrad, R. (1977). Lip-reading by deaf and hearing children. *British Journal of Educational Psychology, 47,* 138–148.
8. Cornett, O. (1985). Diagnostic factors bearing on the use of cued speech with hearing-impaired children. *Ear and Hearing, 6,* 33–35.
9. Nicholls, G., and Ling, D. (1981). Cued speech and the reception of spoken language. *Journal of Speech and Hearing Research, 25,* 262–269.
10. Carmel, S. (1982). *International hand alphabet charts* (2nd ed.). Rockville, MD: Author.
11. Scouten, E. (1942). *A revaluation of the Rochester Method.* Rochester, NY: The Alumni Association of the Rochester School for the Deaf.
12. Goldin-Meadow, S., and Mylander, C. (1984). Gestural communication in deaf children: The effects and noneffects of parental input on early language development. *Monographs of the Society for Research in Child Development, 49.*
13. Lane, H. (1976). *The wild boy of Aveyron.* Cambridge, MA: Harvard University Press.
14. Klima, E., and Bellugi, U. (1979). *The signs of language.* Cambridge, MA: Harvard University Press.

15. Wilbur, R. (1979). *American Sign Language and sign systems.* Baltimore: University Park Press.
16. Gustason, G., Pfetzing, D., and Zawolkow, E. (1972). *Signing exact English.* Silver Spring, MD: National Association of the Deaf.
17. Baldwin, R., and Campbell, M. (1982). Individual educational planning and Public Law 94-142. In D. Sims, G. Walter, and R. Whitehead (Eds.), *Deafness and communication* (pp. 199–208). Baltimore: Williams & Wilkins, p. 199.
18. Strauss, K. (1985). Federal legislation. *Gallaudet Today, 15,* 31–34.
19. *Grove City College v. Bell* (465 US 555, 1984).
20. National Center for Law and the Deaf. (1985). *Educating the hearing impaired child: A legal perspective.* Paper prepared by the staff of the National Center for Law and the Deaf, Washington, DC: Gallaudet College.
21. *Hendrick Hudson Central School District v. Rowley* (102, S. Ct. 3034, 1982).
22. DuBow, S., and Geer, S. (1984, January). Special education law since Rowley. *Clearinghouse Review,* 1001–1007.
23. National Center for Law and the Deaf. (1982). *Analysis of the Rowley decision.* Paper prepared by the staff of the National Center for Law and the Deaf, Washington, DC: Gallaudet College.
24. Allen, R., and Osborn, T. (1984). Academic integration of hearing-impaired students: Demographic, handicapping, and achievement factors. *American Annals of the Deaf, 129,* 100–113.
25. Trybus, R. (1978). What the Stanford Achievement Test has to say about the reading abilities of deaf children. In H. Reynolds and C. Williams (Eds.), *Proceedings of the Gallaudet Conference on Reading in Relation to Deafness* (pp. 213–221). Washington, DC: Gallaudet College.
26. Lenneberg, E. (1967). *Biological foundations of language.* New York: John Wiley & Sons.
27. Mayberry, R., and Fischer, S. (1985). *Sign processing in sentences: The effect of length of experience.* Unpublished manuscript.
28. Mayberry, R., Fischer, S., and Hatfield, N. (1983). Sentence repetition in American Sign Language. In J. Kyle and B. Woll (Eds.), *Language in sign: An international perspective* (pp. 206–214). London: Croom Helm.
29. Mayberry, R., and Eichen, E. (1985). *Points and signs in memory for American Sign Language: The effect of age of acquisition.* Paper presented at the Annual Convention of the American Speech, Language and Hearing Association, Washington, DC, November.
30. Mayberry, R., and Eichen, E. (1986). [Early language and sign language comprehension]. Research in progress.
31. Mayberry, R., and Tuchman, S. (1985). Memory for sentences in

ASL: The influence of age of first learning. In W. Stokoe and V. Volterra (Eds.), *Proceedings of the III. International Symposium on Sign Language Research* (pp. 120–125). Silver Spring, MD: Linstok Press.

32. Newport, E. (1984). Constraints on learning: Studies in the acquisition of American Sign Language. *Papers and Reports on Child Language Development, 23,* 1–22.

33. Frishberg, N. (1975). Arbitrariness and iconicity: Historical change in American Sign language. *Language, 51,* 696–719.

34. Bellugi, U., and Fischer, S. (1972). A comparison of sign language and spoken language. *Cognition, 1,* 173–200.

35. Marmor, G., and Petitto, L. (1979). Simultaneous communication in the classroom: How well is English grammar represented? *Sign Language Studies, 23,* 99–136.

36. Wodlinger-Cohen, R. (1986, June). *The manual representation of speech by deaf children, their mothers, and their teachers.* Paper presented at the Conference on Theoretical Issues in Sign Language Research, Rochester, NY.

37. Mayberry, R., and Wodlinger-Cohen, R. (1986). [Development of written and sign language processing skills]. Research in progress.

38. Conrad, R. (1979). *The deaf school child.* London: Harper & Row.

39. Gaines, R., and Yongxin, P. (1985). Chinese deaf children's reading skills and signing skills. In W. Stokoe and V. Volterra (Eds.), *Proceedings of the III. International Symposium on Sign Language Research* (pp. 91–100). Silver Spring, MD: Linstok Press.

40. Trybus, R., and Karchmer, M. (1977). School achievement scores of hearing impaired children: National data on achievement status and growth patterns. *American Annals of the Deaf Directory of Programs and Services, 122,* 62–69.

41. Madden, R., Gardner, E., Rudman, H., Karlsen, B., and Merwin, J. (1982). *The Stanford Achievement Test for Use with Hearing Impaired Students.* New York: Hart Brace Jovanovich.

CHAPTER 9

Outcomes: Deaf People and Work

McCay Vernon

I f we were to take a criterion and use it as a standard by which to evaluate how the service delivery system functions for deaf people, that criteria would be employment. There is no better measure of the value of education, vocational rehabilitation, employment agencies, and other dimensions of human services to deaf people than what happens to the deaf in the world of work. If deaf people are working productively it means that tax dollars spent to prepare them for employment have represented an investment for society, not an expense.

This chapter will first examine work in a broad psychological cultural sense. Second, the place of the deaf person in the world of work will be described, partly to determine the extent to which the money spent on deaf children and adults is an expense or an investment. Finally, issues surrounding deaf workers and future trends in employment will be considered.

THE SIGNIFICANCE OF WORK

Social planners, philosophers, and scholars who have addressed the fundamental issues of human life have seen work as playing a major role in individual adjustment and in the success and failure of societies throughout history. In order to set a frame of reference to discuss deaf people and work, I will examine how some of these thinkers have perceived work in the framework of society as a whole.

Biopsychologists such as Richard Hernstein and philosophers such as George Bernard Shaw and Frederick Nietzsche have seen work as a form of social Darwinism or social evolution in which economic success is an indicator of survival of the fittest.[1] To them the race of life goes to the swift, and a major aspect of this race is economic. The current controversies over the genetics of intelligence are a substrata underlying this basic perspective. In fact, as the tasks of the workplace become increasing complex, and robotics and automation eliminate most of the simpler routine jobs, we may have a society in which those lacking intelligence and sophisticated training may become anachronisms.

Social thinkers such as Karl Marx and Mao Tse-tung have seen work as so fundamental to personal well-being and to society that they have developed political philosophies around work and the worker. Marx saw work as the fundamental determiner of behavior. Mao said that from work man learns the relationships that exist between people and nature.[2] Marxists and other political theorists generally do not differ on the importance of work; they differ only on how society should treat work and the worker.

Psychology and psychiatry have always agreed with political science on the importance of work. For example, Freud stated, "No other technique for the conduct of life attaches the individual so firmly to reality as laying emphasis on work."[3]

Psychological research has shown that the capacity to work is a cardinal sign of mental health. Prior work history is one of the most powerful predictors of recovery from schizophrenia, drug abuse, alcoholism, and criminal behavior.[4-8] Job satisfaction, job stability, and income are all positively correlated with mental health. By contrast, the percent of one's adult life spent unemployed is negatively correlated with mental health.[1]

Mastery in the workplace reflects ego strength as much as it reflects social conformity, good luck, and intelligence.[1] Work is so tied to self-esteem and meaning in life that people often continue to work long after it is no longer a financial necessity. (This is not to say that we should all be workaholics.)

American executives and labor leaders, by virtue of lack of empathy, have created in American industry an antagonism between workers and employers that threatens to destroy our economic system. In its place may rise the Japanese type of economy, which does place emphasis on empathy between worker and employer.

If we examine chronic unemployment we see that it is not just associated with ignorance, poor education, lack of job skills, and related kinds of deficiencies; at the core of much unemployment is chronic depression and emotional instability.[1]

DEAF PEOPLE IN THE WORLD OF WORK

There is little up-to-date information on deaf people and employment in the United States. The national census on the deaf (Schein and Delk)[8] is over 15 years old. It was the last research of its kind to be done. Over the last decade the employment picture in the industrial world has changed dramatically. I will first review some of the major findings from Schein and Delk's work and then discuss more recent, though less comprehensive, studies.

Unemployment

One of the most surprising findings of Schein and Delk's study was that there was less overall unemployment among deaf people than among the normally hearing. This is a remarkable statistic; it is as hard a fact as one could present as evidence that money spent to educate and rehabilitate deaf people represents an investment, not an expense, to the American taxpayer. The significance of this datum on unemployment must be fully acknowledged if we are to appropriately evaluate the dividend our country realizes on each dollar it puts into education and rehabilitation of deaf people.

Unemployment figures for nonwhite deaf people are much higher than for deaf people in general. They will be discussed separately as part of an examination of hard-core unemployment.

Where Are Deaf People in the Work Force?

Schein and Delk found that most deaf workers are in manufacturing, especially in heavy industries such as steel and automobile production. They tend to be machine operators or assemblers. Some of them work as craftsmen or technicians; a few are professionals. They are seriously underrepresented in personal-service occupations, sales, and management. Schein and Delk believe that the major issue in 1972 was the *under*employment — not *un*employment — of deaf people. They support this position with income data: The average deaf head of a household earns 84 percent as much as the average normally hearing head of a household. Overall, deaf people only earn 72 percent as much as hearing people. Once again, the discrepancies are worse for nonwhite deaf people. Also, the earlier in life the onset of the hearing loss, the lower the income tends to be.

The New Jersey Survey

In 1982, the state of New Jersey completed a survey of its deaf citizens.[9] When we look at these findings, we see that they are consistent with those of Schein and Delk. For example, in New Jersey today, about 30 percent of deaf workers are employed in manufacturing as machine operators, assemblers, and fabricators. Underemployment remains a problem: Many deaf college graduates hold clerical jobs and one was even a garbage collector.

Deaf Graduates of Gallaudet College

A study completed on graduates of Gallaudet College found that 85 percent of Gallaudet graduates were in professional, technical, or managerial jobs.[10] However, on the average they earned less than their hearing counterparts; yearly incomes were $1,000 to $1,500 below those of college graduates in general. The main reason for this income difference appears to be the percent of deaf graduates in teaching or in government employment, where salaries tend to be lower.

When Gallaudet graduates are compared to deaf high school graduates, it is found that their earnings are 50 percent higher. This suggests the value of a college education for deaf people.

The Role of Service Agencies and Other Factors

The Schein and Delk census,[8] the New Jersey survey,[9] and Armstrong's follow-up of Gallaudet graduates[10] indicate that government service agencies play a major role in helping deaf people in the United States gain the employment status they have (which, incidentally, is a far higher employment status than that attained by deaf people in any other country). This is in part due to the number of college programs which are either specifically for deaf students or else have support services for them (e.g., sign language interpreting, note taking, tutoring, etc.).

Deaf clients have a vocational success rate twice that of other disabled groups. In other words, two times more deaf clients are placed in jobs than other disabled persons such as the blind or those with epilepsy. These data are especially significant when it is realized that there is much less per capita investment made for vocational rehabilitation in deaf people than in other groups such as the blind.[8]

What deaf people want from vocational rehabilitation is specific job training, education, or job placement.[8,9] Schein and Delk and the New Jersey survey found that the majority of deaf clients were satisfied with their vocational rehabilitation services. The 20 to 30 percent who were not satisfied complained primarily of poor or slow service, inadequate job placement, and below-standard training facilities. Another major complaint was uninterested, incompetent counselors.[8]

Other isolated but interesting facts were revealed by the New Jersey survey: Eighty-two percent of deaf people have driver's licenses. Fifty-two percent are members of a temple or church. About one half belong to a deaf club. In general, the percentage belonging to a club increases as a function of income. However, employers as a group do not respond favorably to deaf workers.[8] Safety risks, training difficulty, and worker inflexibility are the most common complaints of employers. These problems and employer attitudes are primary contributions to underemployment.

The Hard Core

About 20 to 25 percent of deaf people comprise a hard-core unemployment group[11]: Many are young and from urban areas. A disproportionate number are black or Hispanic. Many receive SSI, welfare, and other forms of government assistance such as Aid to Dependent Children. Crime is high in this group, as are prison costs. Many of these individuals read at a second or third grade level. For some living on welfare, fatherless homes, drug use, and crime are modal behaviors in their communities. This segment of the deaf population may already have become a permanent jobless underclass: Many of these youths will never enter the work force.

This hard core segment of deaf unemployed youth is extremely costly to society both in terms of outright welfare and SSI, and as a result of indirect expenses related to crime, drugs, illegitimate dependent handicapped children, and so forth. Our society has not faced the issue of hard-core unemployed youths in either the deaf or the hearing populations.[11,12] Are we going to continue to pour money down the drain in terms of welfare, SSI, prisons, crimes against innocent citizens, and unwanted dependent children, or are we going to develop programs to solve these problems?

In both financial and human terms, this is one of the more serious issues facing the United States today. The political consequences could threaten the survival of our present form of government by creating a nation of haves and have-nots.[13]

THE FUTURE

What do future trends in the workplace mean for deaf people? The legions of deaf and hearing semiskilled workers who are being forced to leave heavy manufacturing industries will be hard-pressed to find other work.[13-15] For example, arc welding now employs about 750,000 people. Robots will soon do most of this work.[14] A General Electric executive recently said that half of that company's 37,000 assembly workers could be replaced by machines.[14]

Fourteen percent of deaf people used to be employed in printing.[15] Today, however, highly skilled printers with years of experience are actually being paid to quit. The *New York Times* will give an experienced, competent printer with years of service $45,000 cash to quit. One might say, "Wonderful! Why doesn't this deaf printer take the money and go work elsewhere?" Printing has become increasingly automated. Reporters now type their stories using a word processor, cutting out many of the intermediary steps that once existed between report and the press. The linotype has become an anachronism. At a more general level, when skilled union craftspersons are automated out of jobs, they tend to wind up in much lower-paying jobs in service industries or become unemployed.[14]

Deaf workers must look to rapidly expanding fields such as high technology (e.g., computers, bioengineering, and robotics).

Deaf people have successfully moved into the computer field in fairly large numbers, and computer work is taking the place of printing as the most popular high-level field of work for deaf people.[12] Another positive note is that the lower birth rates of the 60s and 70s will mean fewer applicants for lower-level entry jobs in the future.[14]

The worker of today must be geographically, interindustry, and salary mobile. For example, due to changing technology and problems in the auto industry, Flint, Michigan, has about a 30 percent unemployment rate. People are leaving the community en masse. They cannot sell their homes. They are forced to take jobs at much lower salaries, and many are going into entirely different industries.

Implications

For deaf people there are a number of implications that can be drawn from the above. Money invested in deaf people pays dividends both economically and in human terms. To fail to make an adequate investment in the education and training of deaf people would leave the government paying for SSI, welfare, aid to dependent children, crime, and wasted lives.

If we choose to invest in education and training, some basic directions are necessary. Deaf people must be trained for occupations that are in demand. We are not doing that today. For example, almost all schools for the deaf still teach printing, when it is a dead-end field.

If we are going to train deaf people for jobs that are in demand, we have to do a much better job than we are now doing in projecting job needs and the geographic areas where the jobs are to be available. For example, an unemployed machinist in Flint may be able to find out some general information about the supply and demand of machinists, but still has no effective way to know where machinist jobs are to be found.

Also, job training for deaf people must be provided in settings where interpreters or signing instructors are available. The New Jersey survey[9] showed that deaf people have often been sent for training to facilities lacking such services. With the increased level of training required for the new jobs of the future, deaf people will need appropriate supportive services if they are to succeed.

Finally, for the 20 to 25 percent of hard-core deaf (and hearing) unemployed, highly specialized long-term programs are essential.[11,12] To fail to provide these programs is to invite a huge continuing and increasing expense and a political time bomb.

Work is of fundamental psychological importance to human beings, especially deaf people. It is also basic to a society, because without it, there is no productivity, and citizens tend to direct their energies in negative ways such as revolution, crime, and self-destruction.

Historically, this country has invested in the education and training of deaf people. The results have been overwhelmingly positive in both economic and human terms. This can continue to be true if the caliber of training and support services improves, if there is training and placement directly aimed at society's needs occupationally and geographically, and if special programs are provided for the hard-core unemployed.

REFERENCES

1. Vaillant, G. E., and Vaillant, C. O. (1981). Natural history of male psychological health, X: Work as a predictor of mental health. *American Journal of Psychiatry, 138,* 1433–1440.
2. Mao, T. (1961). On practice. *Four essays on philosophy.* Peking: Foreign Language Press.
3. Freud, S. (1961). *Civilization and its discontents (1930) in complete psychological works (Standard ed., Vol. 21,* J. Stachey, Trans. and Ed.). London: Hogarth Press.
4. Costello, R. M. (1975). Alcoholism treatment and evaluation: In search of methods. *International Journal of Addiction, 10,* 251–275.
5. Blueck, S., and Blueck, E. (1943). *Criminal careers in retrospect.* New York: Commonwealth Fund.
6. Stephens, J. H. (1978). Long-term prognosis and follow-up in schizophrenics. *Schizophrenia Bulletin, 4,* 25–47.
7. Vaillant, G. E. (1966). A twelve year follow-up of narcotic addicts, IV: Some characteristic determinants of abstinence. *American Journal of Psychiatry, 123,* 573–584.
8. Schein, J. D., and Delk, M. T. (1974). *The deaf population of the United States.* Silver Spring, MD: National Association of the Deaf.
9. Terzian, A. L., and Saari, M. E. (1982). *Employment and related life experiences of deaf persons in New Jersey.* New Brunswick, NJ: Rutgers State University.
10. Armstrong, D. F. (in press). Income and occupations of deaf former college students.
11. Vernon, M., and Hyatt, C. (1981). How rehabilitation can better serve deaf clients: The problem and some solutions. *Journal of Rehabilitation, 47,* 60–62, 79.

12. Raspberry, W. (1982, 22 March). No miracles — Just jobs. *Washington Post*, A-15.

13. Abelson, P. H. (1982). The revolution in computers and electronics, *Science, 215*, 751–753.

14. Anderson, H., Lampert, H., Young, J., and Malamud, P. (1981, 23 November). Where the jobs are and aren't. *Newsweek*, 88–90.

15. Vernon, M. (1981). The decade of the eighties: Significant trends and developments for hearing impaired individuals. *Rehabilitation Literature, 42*, 2–7.

Author Index

Subject Index

Italic page numbers refer to figures and tables.